Hospital and public Health Safety

Hospital and Public Health Safety

C.Charles

ANMOL PUBLICATIONS PVT. LTD.
NEW DELHI - 110 002 (INDIA)

ANMOL PUBLICATIONS PVT. LTD.
H.O.: 4374/4B, Ansari Road, Darya Ganj
New Delhi-110 002 (India)
Ph.: 23278000, 23261597
B.O.: 1015, Ist Main Road, BSK IIIrd Stage
IIIrd Phase, IIIrd Block
Bangalore - 560 085 (Karnataka)
Ph: 080-41723429, Tel/Fax: 080-2672 3604
Visit us at: www.anmolpublications.com

Hospital and Public Health Safety

First Published, 2008

ISBN 978-81-261-3291-1

PRINTED IN INDIA

Printed at Mehra Offset Press, Delhi.

Contents

Preface

This publication 'Hospital and Public Health Safety' deals with all related issues regarding hospital and public health safety' in modern times. For instance, in USA, the purpose of the Occupational Safety and Health Act of 1970 (Public Law 91596) is to ensure safe and healthful working conditions for every working man and woman in the Nation and to preserve our human resources by providing medical and other criteria that will ensure, insofar as practicable, that no workers will suffer diminished health, functional capacity, or life expectancy as a result of their work experience. The Act authorizes the National Institute for Occupational Safety and Health (NIOSH) to develop and establish recommended occupational safety and health standards, and to conduct the necessary research and experimental programs to develop criteria for new and improved occupational safety and health standards. Although this document does not recommend a new standard, it does present guidelines for reducing the incidence of injury and disease among health care workers. Every effort was made to address all major health and safety hazards that might be encountered in hospitals or other health care centers. The document is not intended to affect patients directly, but implementing the guidelines will generally benefit patient care.

The Hospital Safety Officers conduct hazard surveillance inspections at least once every six months in patient care areas and at least once a year in non-patient care areas. A schedule of inspections is maintained in the office of Hospital Safety as well as a database of areas surveyed and findings. Inspection reports are sent to the cost center managers with copies to appropriate administrators. Written responses from each area surveyed are required. Inspection reports and responses are maintained in binders arranged by building and floor in the office of Hospital Safety. Accidents/incidents involving property damage, personnel, student, or visitor injury and/or occupational illness, are reported in accordance with the Hospital Incident Report Program standard (i178. Incident Report Program) and procedures outlined in the "You and UAB Handbook"(Section 3.2). Hospital Safety reviews incident reports and conducts further investigation when warranted. Incident information is entered into a database for analysis of trends relating to injury type, location, body part, severity and contributing factors. Among the topics of interest to Safety Engineers, Safety Coordinators, Hospital Engineers, Personnel Directors, and Risk Managers are:

— Industrial Hygiene - hospitals are having to provide greater protection for employees and patients from asbestos, chemicals, and environmental conditions.

— Hazard Communication - hospitals should be prepared for this important topic from OSHA and various state right-to-know laws. The material on the topic will help you meet these regulations.

— Hazardous Waste - hospitals now may be classified as small quantity generators and come under EPA regulations as well as a JCAHO standard. Some hazardous wastes are not defined as hazardous waste under these regulations and you should know what they are.

— Disaster Preparation - A section dealing with what is required by JCAHO and NFPA-99. Each plan is different so a checklist is provided to assure that you consider everything as you develop a plan.

— Risk Management - special emphasis is placed on risk management as it applies to medical equipment and its safe use. The policy and procedures for equipment can be used in other areas with slight modification.

— Special Topics - Asbestos, Anesthetic Waste Gas, Ethylene Oxide, Antineoplastic Drugs, AIDS, and Back injuries are hospital safety areas that are given special emphasis.

All the standard safety topics such as job safety analysis, hazard recognition, electrical safety, fire protection and education are covered in depth. For example, the US Food and Drug Administration has received 95 reports of fires involving electrically powered hospital beds since 1993. To help prevent incidents of this kind, they have developed the enclosed lists of safety tips. They apply to all electrically powered healthcare beds. They may be particularly useful for older model beds. One list is intended for the clinical staff and the other for staff responsible for bed maintenance. The Safe Medical Devices Act of 1990 (SMDA) of USA requires hospitals and other user facilities to report deaths and serious injuries associated with the use of medical devices. FDA is interested in additional data on adverse events of fires involving hospital beds. Healthcare providers employed by facilities that are subject to FDA's user facility reporting requirements should follow the reporting procedures established by their facilities.

This publication 'Hospital and Public Health Safety' covers issues and provides answers related to:

— A patient-centered initiative to advance the reliability of healthcare systems worldwide which includes videos, audio cassettes, and CD-ROM training tools.

— Provides integrated technology solutions and consulting services to improve quality and operating performance of emergency departments.

— Provides broad range of safety and quality information for patients, clinicians, and healthcare administrators; online and in print format.

— Supports clinicians in providing safe patient care by designing and testing clinical innovations, technological solutions, and patient safety improvement systems. Research targets the frail elderly and persons with disabilities.

— Promotes development of data standards applicable to the collection, coding and classification of patient safety information. The plan will apply to both adverse event data and errors data.

— Encourages a culture of safety by providing tools that allow health care organizations to communicate, collaborate, improve and share; site includes eCUSP (electronic unit-based patient safety program).

— Provides JCAHO-compliant environment of care safety management and patient safety improvement policies and procedures for health care organizations; resources include online programs and on-site training.

— Provides real-time, secure, patient-centric clinical information in five areas critical for delivering quality care: diagnoses, laboratory results, medications, allergies and immunizations.

—Editor

1

Introduction to Hospital and Public Health Safety

PROMOTING A CULTURE OF SAFETY

In a number of high hazard organisations, where the risk of error involves dire consequences, leaders manage for safe, reliable performance. As a result, the term *High Reliability Organisation* has been coined to describe organisations with exemplary track records of safety: aviation, chemical manufacturing, shipping, nuclear power production, and the military. This concept is rooted in the analyses of errors that reveal organisational failures, along with technical failures (related to system performance) and human limitations (related to human behaviour).

Theories about antecedents to accidents abound but major schools of thought include Reason's belief that a number of latent factors embedded in organisational systems can align and result in accidents, and Rasmussen's approach to categorizing the different sources of error that interact with latent factors to produce accidents. Another school of thought, developed by Charles Perrow and first publicized shortly after the Three Mile Island nuclear accident, *Normal Accident Theory*, emphasizes the ever-present possibility of accidents in organisations that exhibit complexity and "tight coupling" of processes and the inevitability of accidents.

Normal Accident Theory stands somewhat in opposition to *High Reliability Theory*, which holds that accidents can be prevented through organisational design and management. Scott Sagan's analysis of the nuclear weapons industry, addressing the question of why there has never been an 'accidental' nuclear war, represents a fascinating investigation of a test case for these two schools of thought. Despite the obvious apparent confirmation of the *High Reliability Theory* perspective (i.e., such an accident has thankfully never occurred), Sagan uncovers a surprising amount of evidence that also seems to confirm the *Normal Accident* perspective.

Regardless of the underlying theory, healthcare is vulnerable to error. The application of safety promotion theories utilized to positive effect in other high hazard organisations are being considered for healthcare, where "accidents" tend to occur one person at a time instead of in sweeping disasters. Attention to organisational issues of structure, strategy and culture may be a promising direction for medicine. Although organisational elements are intertwined and must be aligned for optimum performance this chapter focuses on the culture component, especially "safety cultures." Following a description of the prevailing models of culture and safety, we review approaches that both medical and non-medical industries have used to promote a culture of safety. On the medical side, the discussion is limited to the Veterans Health Administration's comprehensive safety initiative. On the non-medical side, specific methods other high reliability industries have applied to promote a safety culture, including a behaviour-based industry approach, are reported.

Organisational Culture

Helmreich defines culture as "a complex framework of national, organisational, and professional attitudes and values within which groups and individuals function." Corporate culture is often referred to as the glue that holds an organisation together, and is therefore assumed to be a contributor to organisational performance by socializing workers in a way that increases commitment to the goals of the entity. As such, it embodies the philosophy of senior leaders, which is translated into, and affects the behaviours of employees. Although some schools of thought focus on the role of leaders of an organisation (board members and executives), others note that middle management likely plays a substantial role as well, conveying the culture to front-line workers in any organisation, as evidenced by studies of the effective use of total quality management. The power of culture often goes unrecognized, since employees may assume that the dominant paradigm is simply "the way we do things here."

Safety Culture

While an exact definition of a safety culture does not exist, a recurring theme in the literature is that organisations with effective safety cultures share a constant commitment to safety as a top-level priority, which permeates the entire organisation. More concretely, noted components include: 1) acknowledgment of the high risk, error-prone nature of an organisation's activities, 2) blame-free environment where individuals are able to report errors or close calls without punishment, 3) expectation of collaboration across ranks to seek solutions to vulnerabilities, and 4) willingness on the part of the organisation to direct resources to address safety concerns. Based on extensive field work in multiple organisations, Roberts et al have observed several common, cultural values in reliability enhancing organisations: "interpersonal responsibility; person centeredness; [co-workers] helpful and supportive of one another; friendly, open sensitive personal relations; creativity; achieving goals, strong feelings of credibility; strong feelings of interpersonal trust; and resiliency."

Culture Surveys

The aspect of organisational safety culture that may be visible or measurable is sometimes referred to as the safety "climate," which includes management systems, safety systems, and individual attitudes and perceptions. Healthcare organisations are now adapting safety culture and climate surveys from other industries to benchmark and identify potential deficiencies in their unique safety culture. Kaiser Permanente, the oldest and largest not-for-profit health maintenance organisation in the United States, has administered an executive attitudes and beliefs survey to identify perceptions of patient safety for the purposes of planning and measurement (written communication, February 2001, Suzanne Graham). The VA Palo Alto Patient Safety Center of Inquiry and Stanford University's Center for Health Policy/Center for Primary Care and Outcomes Research are conducting a patient safety culture survey that builds on past work by Gaba and collaborators. The survey includes items on production pressures and safety consequences, and draws from several other sources (personal communication, June, 2001, Sara Singer). Spath provides a checklist of elements that healthcare managers can use to identify which cultural elements should be addressed in order to improve safety. Previous work in assessing organisational culture effects on total quality management, and organisational culture in high reliability organisations may also be pertinent to efforts to measure culture and its consequences for patient safety.

Industries Outside Medicine

Promoting a culture of safety has historically been a

priority for the chemical, electrical, food processing, petroleum, plastic, and transportation industries. Since the 1930s, safety managers within various industries have recognized that most occupational injuries have a strong behavioural component, typically rooted in the safety culture. In these settings, behaviour analysis has been used as an approach to solving safety problems. Behavioural analyses typically involve assessing upstream and downstream behaviours associated with the problem, with further analysis as to which behaviours may be modifiable. Once relevant behaviours are identified, a behaviour change intervention is implemented, and behavioural changes are measured. Interventions are customized, and draw upon techniques of behaviour science, organisational development, safety science, and quality. Researchers have shown associations between behaviour-based safety programmes and reduced rates of accidents.

In an extensive field study of three organisations (nuclear aircraft carriers, a nuclear power plant, and the federal agency responsible for air traffic control) whose operations have the potential for widespread harm, Roberts et al proposed several management processes that "cradle" a culture of perfection. One process requires distributing decision making, while having mechanisms that allow decisions to migrate up and down the chain of command as circumstances develop. The mechanism for localizing decision making is often extensive training, while the approach to moving decisions to higher levels is based on management by exception when acceptable operation is in question. Finally, these researchers suggest that both top-level managers and local operators develop a deep understanding of their organisations, and use this "big picture" perspective to provide intuitive judgments when situations arise.

Practice Description

Veterans Health Administration Approach

The Veterans Health Administration (VHA) has implemented a multifaceted safety initiative, which was designed to build a culture of safety and address system failures. The approach consists of 4 major elements: 1) partnering with other safety-related organisations and affiliates to demonstrate a public commitment by leadership, 2) establishing centers to direct safety efforts, 3) improving reporting systems, and 4) providing incentives to healthcare team members and division leaders. These tactics are detailed below. In addition, several specific initiatives were implemented to address problems, such as bar coding of medications and use of computerized medical records.

To demonstrate a public commitment to the importance of patient safety, the VHA leadership founded the *National Patient Safety Partnership*, along with several major health-related organisations (the American Association of Medical Colleges, the American Hospital Association, the American Medical Association, the American Nurses Association, and the Institute for Healthcare Improvement). In addition, key senior management officials sounded the safety message in congressional testimony. The second part of the VHA's approach involved establishing centers dedicated to the promotion of patient safety. The first of these was the *National Center for Patient Safety*, which directs patient safety efforts for the VHA at a national level. The Director of the Center oversees patient safety efforts for the entire VHA health system and is a recognized authority. Subsequently, four Patient Safety Centers for Inquiry were funded, which are primarily responsible for safety-related research and development. Specifically, the centers are responsible for identifying problems in the patient care process, implementing corrective measures, and studying effects. Currently, one of these centers is studying safety cultures in healthcare organisations. Finally, the *VHA's Virtual Learning Center* contributes to the safety initiative by allowing VHA facilities to share lessons learned. Additional information, such as training, educational programmes, alerts, and advisories are planned.

The third major component of the VHA's initiative involves *incentives* aimed at improving safety. There are two types of incentives offered: 1) the "carrot," which is a monetary award of up to $5000 for individuals and teams that develop approaches to improve safety issues; and 2) the "stick," which is a performance expectation imposed on leaders to improve patient safety. Leaders of the VHA's 22 regional networks must demonstrate involvement in safety-promoting activities, or be subject to consequences, including possible termination of employment. The primary objective of this incentive is to align regional and national leaders' goals.

Last, the VHA has implemented a two-pronged system for capturing adverse events. The first of these systems, the *Patient Safety Event Registry*, mandates reporting of adverse events and "close calls" occurring within the system. Before implementing the Patient Safety Event Registry, regional review of event cases was sporadic. After implementation, event data is systematically shared both regionally and nationally. The second of the systems, the *voluntary reporter identity system*, was developed in conjunction with the National Aeronautics and Space Administration, and allows for anonymous event reporting. It is intended that the use of both reporting systems will together provide a more comprehensive picture of safety management than would be possible with one system alone.

Behaviour-based Safety Programmes

Outside of medicine, the objective of behaviour-based safety interventions is to reduce incidents by managing at-risk behaviours of the organisation and work teams. An approach described by Krause and colleagues consisted of safety assessments, steering committee formation, development of checklists of well-specified critical behaviours related to safety, observer training regarding the critical behaviours, observation and feedback. These steps, somewhat analogous to aspects of crew resource management training approaches, most likely reflect an active safety culture. The Krause study assessed the effectiveness of behavioural safety initiatives in reducing accidents in 229 facilities in various industries, including chemical, electrical, food, plastic, petroleum, transportation, service, and paper manufacturers. The study used an interrupted time series design with the participating industrial sites. Event rates after implementation of the behavioural programme were compared with the Occupational Safety and Health Administration (OSHA) recordable illness/injury rates. Of the 229 participating sites, 73 provided necessary data (others were excluded either because they failed to provide OSHA illness/ injury rates or results of the behavioural initiative). Compared with baseline, the behavioural initiative resulted in an average 26% improvement in targeted safety behaviours during the first year, which rose to 69% by the fifth year.

Prevalence and Severity of the Target Safety Problem

There is no known information about the prevalence of medical error emanating from cultural/organisational problems in healthcare. Culture is known to contribute to the occurrence of errors and accidents. Its contribution relative to other causal factors is unknown, but likely to vary, depending on the type of accident and work environment. The aviation industry attributes its successful safety record in part to analysis of near miss and accident reports. These types of analyses are only possible if the culture supports reporting of errors. Culture changes may, in fact, have their greatest impact on "underground" (unreported) errors, which are extremely difficult to quantify.

Opportunities for Impact

Although no data from ongoing surveys has yet emerged to permit us to accurately quantify safety culture penetration, we nonetheless speculate based on anecdotal evidence that healthcare organisations have plenty of room for improvement. A number of observers have noted large-scale obstacles to promotion of safety culture within healthcare: a pervasive *culture of blame* that impedes acknowledgment of error, and *professional "silos"* that offer unique challenges to changing any universal aspect of healthcare, including culture.

Even before the Institute of Medicine's pivotal *To Err is Human* report was delivered to the public, promoting a safety culture within healthcare had received widespread attention. The Institute for Healthcare Improvement's Web site features a report "Reducing Medical Errors and Improving Patient Safety: Success Stories from the Front Lines of Medicine." It includes articles about the transformation of culture at the prestigious Dana-Farber Cancer Institute after a highly publicized chemotherapy overdose in 1994, which resulted in the death of a patient. Another article in the same series highlighted the major steps, including cultural change, as noted above, taken by leaders of the nation's largest healthcare provider—the Veterans Affairs Healthcare System—after fatal medical errors were reported by the media.

Comment

Measuring the impact of culture on safety-related outcomes is challenging. Culture is a complex and abstract construct that must be inferred from behaviours, and analysis often relies on self-reported data. Research continues to develop a working model of safety culture that permits measurement of several connected concepts: individuals' perceptions and attitudes about safety, individuals' observable safety behaviours, and an organisation's safety management system as evidenced by its policies and management styles. The relative impact of each of these measures on outcomes is another layer of ongoing research.

Although some data support the effectiveness of the entire VHA initiative in improving safety, there are no direct data supporting the effect of promoting a culture of safety. The use of incentives to reward safety-promoting behaviour and publicly demonstrating a commitment to safety are approaches that could be applied in both large and small healthcare settings. The VHA's reporting system will likely be watched, and potentially adapted by large providers who have inconsistent and/or insufficient reporting of safety problems at local, regional, and national levels.

The evidence presented by Krause provides compelling support for the effectiveness of behaviour-based safety programmes in a wide range of industrial settings. Although this exact approach has not been evaluated in healthcare environments, its emphasis on promoting safety culture seems applicable to patient care environments.

As noted in *To Err is Human*, researchers who have studied organisations with a strong safety culture believe that it is "the most critical underlying feature of their accomplishments." Although the nature of the evidence is based on field studies and other methods not typical of medical evidence, it is considered compelling by a number of experts from organisational and other social sciences. At this point, promoting a culture of safety remains surprisingly unexplored in healthcare settings, where the risks of error are high. Further research in this area is warranted, though the threshold for evidence may need a different yardstick than is typically applied in medicine.

Checklist of Elements that Contribute to a Patient-safe Environment

— All people acknowledge that top management provides essential patient safety improvement leadership.

— The organisation has clearly defined patient safety polices.

— All people can explain the organisation's patient safety policies.

— All people are involved in developing patient safety goals, and everyone can explain desired results and measures.

— All people are actively involved in identifying and resolving patient safety concerns.

— All people can explain how their personal performance affects patient safety.

— All people believe they have the necessary authority and resources to meet their responsibilities for patient safety.

— Patient safety performance for all people is measured against goal, clearly displayed, and rewarded.

— A comprehensive review of patient safety is conducted annually, and there is a process in place that drives continuous improvement.

— Regular workplace hazard analyses are conducted to identify patient safety improvement opportunities. The results are used to make changes in patient care activities.

— All people are empowered to correct patient safety hazards as they are identified.

— A comprehensive system exists for gathering information on patient safety hazards. The system is positive, rewarding, and effective, and people use it.

— All people are fully aware of patient incident trends, causes, and means of prevention.

— All injury-producing patient incidents and significant "near misses" are investigated for root cause, with effective preventive actions taken.

— All people who operate patient care equipment are trained to recognize maintenance needs and perform or request timely maintenance.

— All people know immediately how to respond to an emergency because of effective planning, training, and drills.

— Facilities are fully equipped for emergencies; all necessary systems and equipment are in place and regularly tested; and all people know how to use equipment and communicate during emergencies.

— Ergonomics experts are provided when needed and are involved in patient safety assessment and training.

— All supervisors/managers assist in patient safety workplace analyses, ensure physical protections, reinforce training, enforce discipline, and can explain how to provide safe patient care.

DRAWING ON SAFETY PRACTICES FROM OUTSIDE HEALTHCARE

The medical profession's previous inattention to medical error, along with other publicized deficiencies (such as a notable lag in adopting sophisticated information technologies) have invited unfavourable comparisons between healthcare and other complex industries. The first of the two recent Institute of Medicine (IOM) reports on the quality of healthcare in America, *To Err is Human: Building a Safer Health System*, states that "healthcare is a decade or more behind other high-risk industries in its attention to ensuring basic safety." Consequently, one of the goals of this project was to search these other industries for evidence-based safety strategies that might be applied to healthcare.

The relatively short timeline of this project necessitated a focused approach to the search for potentially applicable patient safety practices from non-healthcare writings. Fortunately, many relevant practices have received at least some analysis or empirical study in the healthcare literature. As a practical solution we present original articles from outside healthcare as foundational and background material, rather than as a primary source of evidence. Specific topics and practices reviewed in *Making Healthcare Safer* that clearly derive from fields outside healthcare include:

— Incident reporting.

— Root cause analysis.

— Computerized physician order entry and decision support as a means of reducing medication errors.

— Automated medication dispensing systems.

— Bar coding technology to avoid misidentification errors.

— Aviation-style preoperative checklists for anesthesia equipment.
— Promoting a "culture of safety".
— Crew resource management, a model for teamwork training and crisis response modeled after training approaches in aviation.
— Simulators (of patients or clinical scenarios) as a training tool.
— Human factors theory in the design of medical devices and alarms.

Many readers may still wonder at the relative paucity of safety practices drawn from non-healthcare sources. While the headline-grabbing assessments of medicine's safety have been criticized by researchers and likely overstate the hazard to patients, it is undeniable that some industries, most notably commercial aviation, have safety records far superior to that of healthcare. One issue we faced in compiling this evidence-based review was the extent to which specific practices could be identified as playing a direct and measurable role in this achievement. Interestingly, the same issue—ascertaining a causative variable—arose in reviewing the literature on anesthesia, likely the one field of medicine with a safety record that rivals aviation's.

Significant complications attributable to anesthesia have decreased to the point that major morbidity and mortality are now too rare to serve as practical endpoints for measuring the quality of anesthesia care, even in large multicenter studies. In attempting to account for this decrease, however, it is very difficult to find evidence supporting a causative role for even the most plausible candidates, such as widely utilized intraoperative monitoring standards. In other words, while the field of anesthesia has clearly made tremendous strides in improving patient safety over the past 50 years, it is hard to discern a particular, isolated practice that accounts for the clear and dramatic secular change in its safety. While at one level, a pragmatist might argue, "who cares, as long as it's safe," trying to adopt the lessons of anesthesia (or for that matter aviation) to the rest of healthcare is made more challenging by tenuous causality.

Some might argue that, rather than pinpointing specific practices to embrace from other industries, healthcare institutions should emulate organisational models that promote safety in complex, high-risk industries that manage to operate with high reliability. Analysis of detailed and interesting case studies have fueled a school of thought known as *high reliability theory*, whose proponents suggest a number of organisational features that likely reduce the risk of "organisational accidents" and other hazards. A cogently argued alternative position, often called *normal accident theory*, questions not only these prescriptions for organisational change, but fundamentally challenges the idea of high reliability in certain kinds of complex, "tightly coupled" organisations. These competing schools of thought offer interesting and valuable insights into the ways that organisational strategies foster safety, while cautioning about the ever-present threat of new sources of error that come with increasingly complex human and technical organisations. Unfortunately, this rich literature does not permit ready synthesis within the framework of evidence-based medicine, even using the less stringent standards we adopted in evaluating non-medical literature..

Even the more engineering-oriented of the disciplines with potential relevance to patient safety yielded a surprising lack of empirical evaluation of safety practices. For instance, numerous techniques for "human error identification" and "error mode prediction" purport to anticipate important errors and develop preventive measures prospectively. Their basic approach consists of breaking down the task of interest into component processes, and then assigning a measure of the likelihood of failure to each process. Many of the techniques mentioned in the literature have received little detailed description and few have received any formal validation (e.g., by comparing predicted failures modes with observed errors). Even setting aside demands for validation, the impact of applying these techniques has not been assessed. Total quality management and continuous quality improvement techniques were championed as important tools for change in healthcare based on their presumed success in other industries, but evaluations of their impact on healthcare have revealed little evidence of success.

In the end, we are left with our feet firmly planted in the middle of competing paradigms. One argues that an evidence-based, scientific approach has served healthcare well and should not be relaxed simply because a popular practice from a "safer" industry sounds attractive. The other counters that medicine's slavish devotion to the scientific and epidemiologic method has placed us in a patient safety straightjacket, unable to consider the value of practices developed in other fields because of our myopic traditions and "reality."

We see the merits in both arguments. Healthcare clearly has much to learn from other industries. Just as physicians must learn the "basic sciences" of immunology and molecular biology, providers and leaders interested in making healthcare safer must learn the "basic sciences" of organisational theory and human factors engineering. Moreover, the "cases" presented on rounds should, in addition to classical clinical descriptions, also include the tragedy of the Challenger and the successes of Motorola. On the other hand, an unquestioning embrace of dozens of promising practices from other fields is likely to be wasteful, distracting, and potentially dangerous. We are drawn to a dictum from the Cold War era—"Trust, but verify."

Is the Patient at Increased Risk for Unsafe Driving?

In this study, we will discuss the first step of the *Physician's Plan for Older Drivers' Safety* (PPODS). In particular, we will provide you with a strategy for answering the question, "Is this patient at risk for medically impaired driving?"

To answer this question, first—

Observe the Patient Throughout the Encounter

Careful observation is often the initial step in diagnosis. As you observe the patient, be alert to:

— Poor hygiene and grooming

— Difficulty walking or getting into and out of chairs

— Difficulty with visual tasks

— Difficulty with attention, memory and comprehension

In the example above, Mr. Phillips has difficulty walking and seeing the room numbers. This raises the question of whether he can handle vehicle foot pedals properly or see well enough to drive safely.

Be Alert to Red Flags in the Patient's History, List of Medications, and Review of Systems

As you take the patient's history, be alert to 'red flags'—any medical condition, medication or symptom that can impair driving skills, either through acute effects or chronic functional deficits. For example, Mr. Evans in his study presents with lightheadedness associated with atrial fibrillation. This is a red flag, and he should be counseled to cease driving until control of heart rate and symptoms has been achieved. Similarly, Mr. Bales' acute myocardial infarction is a red flag. Prior to his discharge from the hospital, his physician should counsel him about driving according to the recommendations.

Counseling the Driver in the Inpatient Setting

When caring for patients in the inpatient setting, it can be all too easy for physicians to forget about driving. In a survey of 290 stroke survivors who were interviewed 3 months to 6 years post-stroke, fewer than 35% reported receiving advice about driving from their physicians, and only 13% reported receiving any type of driving evaluation. While it is possible that many of these patients suffered such extensive deficits that both the patient and physician assumed that it was unlikely for the patient to drive again, patients should still receive driving recommendations from their physician.

Counseling for inpatients may include recommendations for permanent driving cessation, temporary driving cessation, or driving assessment and rehabilitation when the patient's condition has stabilized. Such recommendations are intended to promote the patient's safety and, if possible, help the patient regain his/her driving abilities.

Health Risk Assessment

A health risk assessment is a series of questions intended to identify potential health and safety hazards in the patient's behaviours, lifestyle, and living environment. A health risk assessment may include questions about, but not limited to—

— Physical activity and diet

— Dental hygiene
— Use of safety belts
— Presence of smoke detectors and fire extinguishers in the home
— Presence of firearms in the home
— Episodes of physical or emotional abuse

The health risk assessment is tailored to the individual patient or patient population. For example, a pediatrician may ask the patients' parents about car seats, while a physician who practices in a warm-climate area may ask about the use of hats and sunscreen. Similarly, a physician who sees older patients may ask about falls, injuries, and driving.

Mr. Phillips does not have any acute complaints, but his medical history is filled with red flags. His macular degeneration may prevent him from seeing well enough to drive safely. His osteoarthritis may make it difficult for him to operate vehicle controls or turn to view traffic. Regarding his hypertension, diabetes, and congestive heart failure, does he experience any end-organ damage, sensory neuropathies, or cognitive decline that may affect his driving ability? Could any of his medications impair his driving performance?

Keep in mind that many prescription and non-prescription medications have the potential to impair driving skills, either by themselves or in combination with other drugs. Older patients generally take more medications than their younger counterparts and are more susceptible to their central nervous system effects. Whenever you prescribe one of these medications or change its dosage, counsel your patient on its potential to impair driving safety. You may also recommend that your patient undergo formal assessment of function (the next step in PPODS) while he/she is on the medication.

The review of systems can reveal symptoms that may interfere with the patient's driving ability. For example, loss of consciousness, feelings of faintness, memory loss, and muscle weakness all have the potential to endanger the driver.

Perhaps the most glaring red flag of all is the patient's or family member's concern. If your patient asks, "Am I safe to drive?" (or if a family member expresses concern), find out the reason for the concern. Has the patient had any recent crashes or near-misses, or is he/she losing confidence due to declining functional abilities?

Please note that age alone is not a red flag! While many people experience a decline in vision, cognition, and motor skills as they grow older, people experience functional changes at different rates and to different degrees.

Ask about Driving During the Social History/Health Risk Assessment.

If a patient's presentation and/or the presence of red flags lead you to suspect that he/she is at risk for medically impaired driving, the next step is to ask whether he/she drives. You can do this by incorporating the following questions into the social history or health risk assessment:

— "How did you get here today?"

— "Do you drive?"

If your patient drives, then his/her driving safety should be addressed. For acute events, this generally involves counseling the patient. For example, Mr. Bales should be counseled to temporarily cease driving for a certain period of time after his myocardial infarction. If Mr. Phillips is started on a new medication, he should be counseled about the side effects and their potential to impair driving performance.

For chronic conditions, on the other hand, driving safety is addressed by formally assessing the functions that are important for driving. This is the next step in PPODS.

Please note that many chronic medical conditions have both chronic and acute effects. For example, a patient with insulin-dependent diabetes may experience acute episodes of hypoglycemia in addition to chronic complications such as diabetic retinopathy. In this case, the physician should counsel the patient to avoid driving during acute episodes of hypoglycemia and to keep candy or glucose tablets within reach in the car at all times. The physician should also recommend formal assessment of function if the patient shows any signs of functional decline.

If your patient does not drive, you may wish to ask if he/she ever drove, and if so, why he/she stopped driving. If your patient voluntarily stopped driving due to medical reasons that are potentially treatable, you may be able to help him/her return to safe driving. In this case, formal assessment of function can be performed to identify specific areas of concern and measure the patient's improvement with treatment.

Gather Additional Information

To gain a better sense of your patient as a driver, ask questions specific to driving. The answers to these questions can help you determine the level of intervention that is needed.

If a collateral source such as a family member is available at the appointment or bedside, consider addressing your questions to both the patient and the collateral source. If this individual has had the opportunity to observe the patient's driving, his/her feedback may be valuable.

Questions to ask include:

— "How much do you drive?" (or "How much does [patient] drive?")
— "Do you usually have any passengers?"
— "Do you have any problems when you drive?" (Ask specifically about day and night vision, ease of operating the steering wheel and foot pedals, confusion, and delayed reaction to traffic signs and situations.)
— "Do you think you are a safe driver?"
— "Do you ever get lost while driving?"
— "Have you gotten any tickets in the past two years?"
— "Have you had any near-misses or crashes in the past two years?"

Understand Your Patient's Mobility Needs

At this time, you can also ask about your patient's mobility needs and encourage him/her to begin exploring alternative transportation options. Even if alternative options are not needed at this time, it is wise for the patient to plan ahead in case he/she ever retires from driving. Some questions you can use to initiate the conversation include:

— "How do you usually get around? Does this work well for you?"
— "If your car ever broke down, how would you get around?"

Encourage your patients to plan a safety net of transportation options by telling them, "Mobility is very important for your physical and emotional health. If you were ever unable to drive for any reason, I'd want to be certain that you could still make it to your appointments, pick up your medications, go grocery shopping, and visit your friends." In the event that your patient must retire from driving, the transition from driver to non-driver status will be less traumatic if he/she has already created a transportation plan. The handout in Appendix B, *Getting By Without Driving*, can help your patient get started.

RED FLAGS FOR MEDICALLY IMPAIRED DRIVING

Acute Events

Prior to hospital or emergency department discharge, patients and appropriate caregivers should be counseled as needed regarding driving restrictions and future assessment and rehabilitation. Acute events that can impair driving performance include:

— Acute myocardial infarction

— Acute stroke and other traumatic brain injury

— Syncope and vertigo

— Seizure

— Surgery

— Delirium from any cause

Patient's or Family Member's Concern

Has your patient approached you with the question, "Am I safe to drive?" (Alternatively, a family member may express concern about the patient's driving safety.) If so, find out the cause of concern. Note that age alone does not predict driving fitness—function, not age, is the determining factor. Ask for specific causes of concern, such as recent crashes, near-misses, traffic tickets, becoming lost, poor night vision, forgetfulness, and confusion.

Medical History: Chronic Medical Conditions

Patients may require formal assessment to determine the impact of these conditions on their level of function:

— *Diseases affecting vision*, including cataracts, diabetic retinopathy, macular degeneration, glaucoma, retinitis pigmentosa, field cuts, and low visual acuity even after correction

— *Cardiovascular disease*, especially when associated with pre-syncope, syncope or cognitive deficits, including unstable coronary syndrome, arrhythmias, congestive heart failure, hypertrophic obstructive cardiomyopathy, and valvular disease

— *Neurologic disease*, including dementia, multiple sclerosis, Parkinson's disease, peripheral neuropathy, and residual deficits from stroke

— *Psychiatric disease*, including mood disorders, anxiety disorders, psychotic illness, personality disorders, and alcohol or other substance abuse

— *Metabolic disease*, including Type I and Type II diabetes mellitus and hypothyroidism

— *Musculoskeletal disabilities*, including arthritis and foot abnormalities

— Chronic renal failure

— *Respiratory disease*, including chronic obstructive pulmonary disease and obstructive sleep apnea

Medical History: Medical Conditions with Unpredictable/ Episodic Events

The patient should be counseled not to drive during any of the following acute events:

— Pre-syncope or syncope

— Angina

— Seizure
— Transient ischemic attack
— Hypoglycemic attack
— Sleep attack or cataplexy

Medications

Many non-prescription and prescription medications have the potential to impair driving ability, either by themselves or in combination with other drugs. Combinations of drugs may affect drug metabolism and excretion, and dosages may need to be adjusted accordingly.

— Anticholinergics
— Anticonvulsants
— Antidepressants
— Antiemetics
— Antihistamines
— Antihypertensives
— Antiparkinsonians
— Antipsychotics
— Benzodiazepenes and other sedatives/anxiolytics
— Muscle relaxants
— Narcotic analgesics
— Stimulants

Review of Systems

The review of systems can reveal symptoms or conditions that may impair driving performance. In addition to further work-up, driving safety should be addressed.

— *General:* fatigue, weakness
— *HEENT:* headache, head trauma, visual changes, vertigo

- *Respiratory:* shortness of breath
- *Cardiac:* chest pain, dyspnea on exertion, palpitations, sudden loss of consciousness
- *Musculoskeletal:* muscle weakness, muscle pain, joint stiffness and pain, decreased range of motion
- *Neurologic:* loss of consciousness, feelings of faintness, seizures, weakness/paralysis, tremors, loss of sensation, numbness, tingling
- *Psychiatric:* depression, anxiety, memory loss, confusion, psychosis, mania

Assessment and Plan

As you formulate a diagnosis/treatment plan for your patient's medical conditions, remember to address driving safety as needed. You may need to counsel your patients about driving when you:

- Prescribe a new medication, or change the dosage of a current medication
- Work up a new-onset disease presentation or treat an unstable medical condition. This includes many of the medical conditions listed above.

LET US BE YOUR SAFETY RESOURCE

The National Safety Council, Greater Omaha Chapter, founded in 1924, is a private, nonprofit, community-based organization and an accredited chapter of the National Safety Council. The Council promotes safety and health by providing programmes, resource services and education to prevent both the personal and economic loss associated with injuries, accidents and health hazards wherever they exist. This mission is unique to the Safety Council in this area. Unintentional injuries are the leading cause of death for people aged 1 to 38 and the 5th cause overall.

The toll of non fatal injuries is also enormous. Each year about 2.6 million Americans are hospitalized for injuries, about 39.6 million people are treated in hospital emergency departments, and about 60.5 million people - nearly one in four seek medical attention or suffer at least one day of activity restriction due to an injury. The economic impact of these fatal and non fatal unintentional injuries amounted to $444.1 billion in 1996. This is about $1,700 per capita, or about $4,500 per household. The Safety Council targets the causes by providing programmes in occupational safety and health, community safety, traffic safety, behind the wheel driver education, and personal accountability or individual behavior choices that impact safety. Participants in all categories of programmes are as diverse as the population of the greater Omaha area. Programmes for the schools, businesses and courts are presented to all populations.

Administration and Staff

The president serves as the chief executive officer of the Council, accountable for overall management and supervision of the organization. Five senior staff and 20 additional staff members with expertise in programme and curriculum development, implementation and evaluation, training, consulting, public relations, marketing, network management, data entry and other programme support, work in these areas of programme emphasis: administration, occupational safety and health, crime reduction, traffic safety and community safety. Fifty part-time instructors teach for the Council.

Staff Directory

Financial Management and Planning

A community based volunteer board of directors oversees the management and financial affairs of the Council.

Reflective of the community, they represent large and small business and labor, education, public safety, health and medical areas, law enforcement, emergency services and the justice system. Quarterly executive committee meetings and quarterly board meetings are held to keep board members current on all developments. Individual committees meet during the interim. A yearly board conference is held to review and refine the mission statement and build upon the continuing long-range strategic plan of the Council.

Seventy six percent of Council revenues are earned through membership dues, safety training, safety materials and conference attendance. Twenty two percent is raised through grants and contributions. All funds are committed to safety and health programmes as follows:

The Council's financial affairs are driven by long-range programme activities and a formal strategic plan. Accountability is maintained through the yearly budgeting process and regular reviews and forecasts.

The Council has an accountant on staff. The accounting system includes standard and accepted policies and procedures, accrual system, and an internal purchasing control system. Computer software provides sophisticated allocation and reporting capabilities. The Council has a yearly audit conducted by an independent Certified Public Accounting firm.

Growth of the Council

In the past 10 years, the membership of Omaha area businesses and corporations has increased from 300 to more than 1000. These members represent almost 300,000 employees all across the state. Through the ripple effect, the Council has the ability to reach 300,000 families. With a family average of 2.63 that equates to almost 789,000 people.

The growth of programmes and services has grown even more rapidly than membership. In this growth, we have reached an increasing number of children, people who work in high risk situations, and have been instrumental in decreasing traffic accidents and injuries.

Annually, that's approximately 50,000 individuals trained in injury prevention - 20,000 of that through programmes addressing safe driving practices in an effort to help reduce the over 40,000 people killed every year in the U.S. in traffic crashes - 10,000 in occupational safety and health and crime reduction programmes - and 20,000 in community safety programmes. Millions of safety messages impressions are disseminated throughout our community through television, radio and print public service announcements and safety awareness programmes conducted in area schools and businesses.

Our success has created its own challenges. The Council moved into larger office and training facilities in 1992. By 1995 we found that the demands for safety assistance required that we again relocate into larger facilities. In January 1999, the Council moved into its own building at 11620 M Circle in Omaha with offices and training facilities designed for our specific needs. The decision was made only after a 4 year search and assessment period that determined the organization must build its own facility and that it could manage the construction debt within its operating budget.

Programme Experience

The Council is recognized nationally among other councils and safety professionals as a leader in meeting the safety and health needs. There are many more programmes available to the businesses, children, families, and workers in this area than in other cities of the US. As a result, businesses in outlying communities have requested and received assistance from the National Safety Council, Greater Omaha Chapter in building their safety programmes.

In addition, the National Safety Council, Greater Omaha Chapter has responded to the safety education and training needs of the community where there were important issues and no other solution. The Council assumed the high school behind-the-wheel driver education programme when the Omaha Public School District could no longer include it in their budget. The Council stepped forward to meet the needs of a City of Omaha ordinance for handgun safety training when carrying of these hand guns required professional safety training. Likewise, the motorcycle safety programme has been a response to the State of Nebraska to train new riders in the correct handling of their cycles.

The Work of the Council

The National Safety Council, Greater Omaha Chapter devotes all of its energies to safety and health — injury reducing, life saving education, consultation and awareness programmes. Our partners are businesses, schools, government, law enforcement, fire fighters, and many more.

The Council also either currently or previously provided strong representation to the following groups: American Society of Safety Engineers, Eastern Nebraska Office on Aging, Fireworks Injury Prevention Coalition, Health and Wellness Consortium, Leadership Omaha, Iowa Western Community College Safety Engineering Technology Advisory Committee, Millard Schools Crime Watch Committee, Omaha Public Schools Familyness Committee and Drug Free School Committee, Nebraska Chapter of American Academy of Pediatrics Safety Committee, Nebraska Injury Prevention Coalition, Nebraska Safe Kids, National Safety Council (NSC) Board of Directors, NSC Chapter and Affiliate Division chairman, NSC Accreditation Review Task Force, NSC

Education Task Force, Omaha 2000 Goal VI Task Force, "Please Be Seated" Coalition, Omaha Metropolitan Medical Response Organization, Project Extra Mile, Workforce Investment Board Youth Council, Public Relations Society of America- Nebraska Chapter, Safe Futures, Safety Patrol Advisory Board, and the Omaha Police Chief's Steering Committee and more.

Traffic Safety

Motor vehicle crashes continue as the leading cause of unintentional fatalities and injuries. The Council provides many defensive driving education programmes both general and specific. NSC Attitudinal Dynamics of Driving, NSC Defensive Driving, and the Handicapped Awareness Programme are education programmes available to individuals in lieu of a fine, court costs and points on their driving record if they receive a citation in surrounding counties.

The Council conducts NSC Defensive Driving - 8 hours for drivers license reinstatement training and point reduction programmes for the state of Nebraska and other defensive driving training for the Douglas and Sarpy County Courts.

Additional work in this area is accomplished through training programmes for specific vehicles such as emergency vehicles, vans, straight trucks as well as experienced driver and mature driver programmes.

The number one cause of death and injury for youth ages 15 to 25 is a traffic crash. Through the Behind the Wheel Driver Education programme, begun in 1992 to reach this population, more than 10,000 youth have learned to drive correctly and safely. The programme is rapidly expanding to meet the needs of more and more young drivers and the graduated licensing law passed in 1998 by the legislature. The Council educated more than 1,500 young drivers in this programme in 2002.

The mileage death rate (death per miles driven) is used as a measurement when discussing some vehicles that are not used as commonly yet are very dangerous. One in particular, motorcycles, cause more than 14 times the mileage death rate for occupants of other types of vehicles. Because of the danger and the growing popularity of motorcycles as a recreational vehicle for families, Motorcycle Safety Training was begun in 1998 under the rules of the National Motorcycle Safety Foundation and the State of Nebraska. Individuals passing the Basic Skills Course do not take the written or driving exam for the Motorcycle Operator's License.

In this same area of injuries and deaths on our highways and byways, the Council provides education through continuing public education and awareness programmes on seat belt use, child safety seats and alcohol use. One of the most important programmes, encourages people to buckle up and drive safe and sober includes strong support efforts from law enforcement.

In 1992 the Council received the first National Safety Council Public Policy Recognition for the Council's work in promoting the safety belt law in Nebraska. And it continues it work with businesses encouraging safety belt use and honoring success through the National Safety Belt Honor Roll.

Community Safety

For children in the 5 to 14 year age group, unintentional injuries claim more than all other diseases combined! In 1997, the Council formed the Safe Kids Coalition which includes most area hospitals, all area school districts, PTA and PTO representation, family service centers, the Omaha

Fire Department and several area businesses. As part of the Safe Kids programmes the Council specifically targets bicycle injuries and sponsors Gear Up Games during Child Safety Week, holds child safety coloring and poster contests and school traffic safety programmes such as Pre-School Traffic Training, Safe Walk to School and Back to School Safely.

Community Awards Recognition is given yearly to individuals and businesses who have provided and promoted positive action in safety and health encouraging others to do the same.

An expansion of bicycle safety programmes in 2000, "Helmets for Kids," brought together groups of bicycle safety advocates under the Safe Kids banner. Providing education, reduced cost bicycle helmets and free helmets for those in need is a continuing goal of the Council led coalition.

In 2000 the Council inaugurated the Child Safety Seat Honor Roll. Honorary Members, those who have provided educational awareness to the broad community and Charter Members, business members who have held child safety seat checks or provided support to those checks were recognized at the 2000 Awards Luncheon. Businesses will be encouraged to become members of the Child Safety Seat Honor Roll by participating in Child Safety Seat education through 3 venues.

From 1992 to 1996, the Council implemented the Operation FireSafe smoke detector programme, in cooperation with the Omaha Fire Division and firefighters throughout the 5 county area that includes western Iowa. Firefighters visited every owner occupied residence in the city and installed free smoke detectors and/or batteries to ensure everyone is protected from fire. Again, in 2000, the Council took a leadership role by providing smoke detectors to all surrounding volunteer departments in the Tri County Mutual Aid Association for installation by the firefighters in homes of those most at risk, the elderly and/or economically disadvantaged.

Support to volunteer departments continues today.

The Click It - Don't Risk It safety belt usage campaign works to get people buckled up. In 2003 Nebraska experienced low usage rate and expanding traffic fatalities.

Nebraska Cares, the Council's child passenger safety education programme, has provided hospital staff education on the safe motor vehicle transportation of all children including premature infants and infants and children with disabilities. Initially the programme provided education to all Nebraska hospitals' nursing staff working with children and helped the hospitals write their child transportation policies. To expand the programme, the Council worked with Emergency Medical Services personnel in the development of grass roots resources for communities across the state. The programme has also focused on child care providers and physicians across the state. Child Passenger Safety Education has changed considerably over the past few years due to liability issues and certification requirements. Still, the Council continues to provide resource information, training and child safety seat checks at no cost to parents and caregivers.

And efforts in 2003 will once again address the integration of child passenger safety into the health care arena. With the input of health care facilities the Council will once again provide education to hospital personnel across the state.

Court Services

Personal Accountability and Safety go hand in hand. The individual behavior choices made by each person directly impacts relationships with others and sets one on the path to destructive or positive life styles that impact the safety of our community. The choices are individual for adults and youth whether to drink, use drugs, pursue a life of violence and crime or be a positive contributing member of society. The path chosen has a direct relationship to potential injury.

The Council educates through special programmes which teach individual decision making skills and development of actual individual cognitive responses. The effect of these programmes ultimately is behavior modification for the benefit of all.

The Minor in Possession programme was developed at the request of Omaha 2000, Goal VI task force. Both parents and teens participate in this programme which is skill building, educational and informative for young adults helping them to develop new skills aimed at resisting status offenses and ultimately makes the choices clear to teens.

Anger Management, juvenile and adult programmes, are those most recently implemented. The Council has received an endorsement from the Dr. Robert Meier, Chair of the Department of Criminal Justice at the University of Nebraska at Omaha. Probationers of many offenses can be helped through programmes of the Council which focus on behavior modification goals. Here is one of the largest growing areas of the population and one which according to the criminal violence trends unless checked will greatly increase injury costs. A programme of the Council, "Living Skills, Making Appropriate Decisions" specifically developed in 1997 for Sarpy County Probation and more recently adopted by Douglas County provides education for this segment of the population.

Other programmes for the courts include the DUI, Driving Under the Influence programme and the National Safety Council Step Forward programme which serves the juvenile offender population.

Occupational Safety and Health

Great progress in injury prevention has been made over the years in occupational safety and health, yet costs to employers continue to be huge. And the cost is not only in workers' compensation but in lost productivity, medical costs, administrative expenses, and time lost by other employees.

The Council targets all of this through numerous safety and health training programmes and consultation programmes for businesses conducted by our occupational safety and health training and consulting staff.

The National Safety Council Advanced Safety Certificate is provided in Omaha as are other certificated programmes including the NSC OSHA Compliance Certificate and the NSC Principles Certificate programme. Individuals receive continuing education units for their training. In 2003, National Safety Council, Greater Omaha Chapter was named an OSHA Training Institute Educational Center as part of a consortium that includes St. Louis University, Kirkwood Community College in Iowa and the Safety Council.

In 1998 the Council was awarded an OSHA grant to provide training for safety and health hazards in the red meat industry with Spanish language emphasis. The programme continues with the development of a training video in English and Spanish, English and Spanish workbooks, facilitators guide and power point presentation available to the meatpacking industry.

The Council previously received an OSHA targeted training grant to assist small businesses in development of their Hazard Communication programme. More than 1,000 small businesses were trained under this programme during 1990 and 1991. Until recently, the Council was the only NSC chapter to receive an OSHA grant. In 1997 under an OSHA grant, the Council translated the Haz Com video and employee manual into 5 languages.

The Eastern Nebraska Health Care Safety Network was organized by the Council in 1983. This group of health care safety directors and human resource and security personnel meets monthly in a sharing network. For many years the Council has recognized workplace successes through the Occupational Safety and Health Awards Programme. In 2003, more than 80 companies were recognized for outstanding programmes. Since 1984 the Council has presented the annual Great Plains Safety and Health Conference and Products Show, which attracts more than 1,500 people for the exposition, seminars and other special events. Other mini-conferences are held throughout the year. In 1999 the Council presented the first Governor's Conference on Drugs and Alcohol in the Workplace.

Community Support is Far Reaching

The achievements of the Safety and Health Council reflect the invaluable support and endorsements of area businesses, local government, police and fire departments and individuals who have generously supported the Council. All of these "members of safety" have trusted their investments for more than 75 years with the Council and continue to do so today.

2

Laboratory and Biosafety Guidelines

CRITERIA FOR IMPLEMENTATION OF CHEMICAL CONTROL MEASURES

RSO's – note and delete: This section does not require extensive tailoring. However, research safety officers for some departments have provided descriptions and floor plans that identify the location of equipment such as fume hoods, biological safety cabinets, glove boxes, showers, eyewashes, fire extinguishers, etc.

Engineering controls, personal protective equipment, hygiene practices, and administrative controls each play a role in a comprehensive laboratory safety program. Implementation of specific measures must be carried out on a case-by-case basis, using the following criteria for guidance in making decisions. Assistance is available from the Department of Environmental Health and Safety.

1. Engineering Controls

(a) Fume Hoods

The laboratory fume hood is the major protective device available to laboratory workers. It is designed to capture chemicals that escape from their containers or apparatus and to remove them from the laboratory environment before they can be inhaled. Characteristics to be considered in requiring fume hood use are physical state, volatility, toxicity, flammability, eye and skin irritation, odor, and the potential for producing aerosols. A fume hood should be used if a proposed chemical procedure exhibits any one of these characteristics to a degree that (1) airborne concentrations might approach the action level (or permissible exposure limit), (2) flammable vapors might approach one tenth of the lower explosion limit, (3) materials of unknown toxicity are used or generated, or (4) the odor produced is annoying to laboratory occupants or adjacent units.

Procedures that can generally be carried out safely outside the fume hood include those involving (1) water-based solutions of salts, dilute acids, bases, or other reagents, (2) very low volatility liquids or solids, (3) closed systems that do not allow significant escape to the laboratory environment, and (4) extremely small quantities of otherwise problematic chemicals. The procedure itself must be evaluated for its potential to increase volatility or produce aerosols.

In specialized cases, fume hoods will contain exhaust treatment devices, such as water wash-down for perchloric acid use, or charcoal or HEPA filters for removal of particularly toxic or radioactive materials.

(b) Safety Shields

Safety shields, such as the sliding sash of a fume hood, are appropriate when working with highly concentrated acids, bases, oxidizers or reducing agents, all of which have the potential for causing sudden spattering or even explosive release of material. Reactions carried out at non-ambient pressures (vacuum or high pressure) also require safety shields, as do reactions that are carried out for the first time or are significantly scaled up from normal operating conditions.

(c) Other Containment Devices

Other containment devices, such as glove boxes or vented gas cabinets, may be required when it is necessary to provide an inert atmosphere for the chemical procedure taking place, when capture of any chemical emission is desirable, or when the standard laboratory fume hood does not provide adequate assurance that overexposure to a hazardous chemical will not occur. The presence of biological or radioactive materials may also mandate certain special containment devices. High strength barriers coupled with remote handling devices may be necessary for safe use of extremely shock sensitive or reactive chemicals. Highly localized exhaust ventilation, such as is usually installed over atomic absorption units, may be required for instrumentation that exhausts toxic or irritating materials to the laboratory environment. Ventilated chemical storage cabinets or rooms should be used when the chemicals in storage may generate toxic, flammable or irritating levels of airborne contamination.

2. Personal Protective Equipment

Bare feet, sandals and open-toed shoes are not permitted in any laboratory. Short pants and short skirts are not permitted in any laboratory, unless covered by a lab coat. Lab coats are strongly encouraged as routine equipment for all laboratory workers. Lab coats are also required when working with select carcinogens, reproductive toxins, substances which have a high degree of acute toxicity, strong acids and bases, and any substance on the OSHA PEL list carrying a "skin" notation. See Appendix B for chemical listings.

Eye protection is required for all personnel and any visitors whose eyes may be exposed to chemical or physical hazards. Side shields on safety spectacles provide some protection against flying particles, but goggles or face shields are necessary when there is a greater than average danger of eye contact with liquids. A higher than average risk exists when working with highly reactive chemicals, concentrated corrosives, or with vacuum or pressurized glassware systems. Contact lenses may be worn under safety glasses, goggles or other eye and face protection. Experts currently believe the benefits of consistent use of eye protection outweigh potential risks of contact lenses interfering with eye flushing in case of emergency. Gloves made of appropriate material are required to protect the hands and arms from thermal burns, cuts, or chemical exposure that may result in absorption through the skin or reaction on the surface of the skin. Gloves are also required when working with particularly hazardous substances where possible transfer from hand to mouth must be avoided. Thus gloves are required for work involving pure or concentrated solutions of select carcinogens, reproductive toxins, substances which have a high degree of acute toxicity, strong acids and bases, and any substance on the OSHA PEL list carrying a "skin" notation.

Since no single glove material is impermeable to all chemicals, gloves should be carefully selected using guides from the manufacturers. General selection criteria are outlined in Prudent Practices, p. 132, and glove selection guides are available on the web . However, glove-resistance to various chemicals materials will vary with the manufacturer, model and thickness. Therefore, review a glove-resistance chart from the manufacturer you intend to buy from before purchasing gloves. When guidance on glove selection for a particular chemical is lacking, double glove using two different materials, or purchase a mulitlayered laminated glove such as a Silvershield or a 4H. Respiratory protection is generally not necessary in the laboratory setting and must not be used as a substitute for adequate engineering controls. Availability of respiratory protection for emergency situations may be required when working with chemicals that are highly toxic and highly volatile or gaseous. If an experimental protocol requires exposure above the action level (or PEL) that cannot be reduced, respiratory protection will be required. Rarely, an experimental situation may potentially involve IDLH (immediately dangerous to life or health) concentrations of chemicals, which will require use of respiratory protection. All use of respiratory protective equipment is covered under the University of Minnesota Respiratory Protection Program.

3. Hygiene Practices

Eating, drinking and chewing gum are all strictly prohibited in any laboratory with chemical, biological or radioactive materials. Researchers must also be careful to restrict other actions (such as applying lip balm or rubbing eyes) which could inadvertently cause exposure to research materials. Consuming alcohol or taking illegal drugs in a research laboratory are strictly prohibited, as such actions potentially endanger the health and safety of not only the user, but everyone in the building. Infractions will be met with serious disciplinary action. Before leaving the laboratory, remove personal protective equipment/clothing (labcoat and gloves) and wash hands thoroughly. Do NOT wear laboratory gloves in public spaces such as hallways and elevators.

4. Administrative Controls

Researchers are strongly encouraged to prioritize research so that work with hazardous chemical, biological or physical agents occurs only during working hours (8 am – 5 pm, Monday through Friday). After-hours work (on nights and weekends) should be restricted to nonhazardous activities such as data analysis and report writing. If hazardous materials must be used at nights or on weekends, ensure that at least one other person is within sight and ear-shot to provide help in an emergency.

Supervisors shall consider the hazards involved in their research, and designate areas, activities, and tasks that require specific types of personal protective equipment as described above.

MANAGEMENT OF CHEMICAL FUME HOODS AND OTHER PROTECTIVE EQUIPMENT

RSO's – note and delete: Each PI should identify the safety equipment to be used in the laboratory, and ensure that all employees are properly trained in its use. Since no two fume hoods operate exactly alike, be sure you and your staff understand the operating principals and use safe operating procedures. Please call Environmental Health and Safety for assistance. The Research Safety Officer should insert the name and phone number of the Facilities Management Zone or Hospital Engineers which serves the laboratories in the department [in the underlined section].

1. Monitoring Safety Equipment

Fume hoods must be monitored daily by the user to ensure that air is moving into the hood. Any malfunctions must be reported immediately to the appropriate Facilities Management zone office. The hood should have a continuous reading device, such as a pressure gauge, to indicate that air is moving correctly. Users of older hoods without continuous reading devices should attach a strip of tissue or yarn to the bottom of the vertical sliding sash. The user must ensure the hood and baffles are not blocked by equipment and bottles, as air velocity through the face may be decreased. DEHS staff will measure the average face velocity of each fume hood annually with a velometer or a thermoanemometer. A record of monitoring results will be made.

Eye washes must be flushed weekly by the user. This will ensure that the eye wash is working, and that the water is clean, should emergency use become necessary. The user should coordinate with [Facilities Management or Hospital Engineers (phone number)] to ensure that emergency showers and eye washes are checked annually. Fire extinguishers will be checked annually by a University contractor. The user is responsible for checking regularly to ensure that other protective equipment is functioning properly. Environmental Health and Safety staff can assist with these evaluations, should assistance be necessary.

General laboratory conditions must be monitored periodically by the users. A generic laboratory audit form is included in Appendix G, and may be tailored for use by individual laboratories. The departmental Research Safety Officer or the University's Chemical Hygiene Officer may also use this form for spot-checks of the laboratories.

2. Acceptable Operating Range

The acceptable operating range for fume hoods is 80 to 150 linear feet per minute, at the designated sash opening (usually 18 inches). If, during the annual check, a hood is operating outside of this range, DEHS staff may request that you check to ensure the baffles are adjusted properly, and that the exhaust slots are not blocked by bottles and equipment. If these adjustments do not help, DEHS staff will report the deficiency to the appropriate Facilities Management zone office for servicing.

3. Maintenance

During maintenance of fume hoods, laboratories must clean out and if necessary, decontaminate the fume hood and restrict use of chemicals to ensure the safety of maintenance personnel. See "Safe Practices During Servicing of Exhaust Systems in Research Facilities" in Appendix E.

4. Training

Training in the appropriate use and care of fume hood systems, showers, eyewashes and other safety equipment must be included in the initial and update training described in this study.

5. New Systems

When new ventilation systems, such as variable air volume exhaust, are installed in University facilities, specific policies for their use will be developed by the Department of Environmental Health and Safety and employees will be promptly trained on use of the new equipment.

RECORD KEEPING, REVIEW AND UPDATE OF LABORATORY SAFETY PLAN

A. Record Keeping

Exposure Evaluation

Any records of exposure evaluation carried out by individual departments (including continuous monitoring systems) will be kept within the department and also sent to the Department of Environmental Health and Safety. Results of exposure evaluations carried out by DEHS will be kept by DEHS and sent to the affected department. Raw data will be kept for one year and summary data for the term of employment plus 30 years.

Medical Consultation and Examination

Results of medical consultations and examinations will be kept by the Boynton Health Service for a length of time specified by the appropriate medical records standard. This time will be at least the term of employment plus 30 years as required by OSHA.

Training

Individual employee training should be recorded on form BA 725A and should be kept in the individual's department or college for five years. These forms may be audited by the University Audit Department.

Fume Hood Monitoring

Data on annual fume hood monitoring will be kept in the Department of Environmental Health and Safety. Fume hood monitoring data are considered maintenance records and as such the raw data will be kept for one year and summary data for 5 years.

B. Review and Update of Laboratory Safety Plan

On an annual basis, this Laboratory Safety Plan will be reviewed and evaluated for effectiveness by the Department of Environmental Health and Safety and updated as necessary. Any changes in the Laboratory Safety Plan will be transmitted to college and departmental research safety officers, who are responsible for carrying out a similar review and modification of their plans, and submitting a revised copy to the Chemical Hygiene Officer.

3

Hospital Investigations and Safety Against Infections

HOSPITAL INVESTIGATIONS: HEALTH HAZARDS

Introduction

Incidence and Casual Factors

As of 1988, 4% of the total U.S. work force was employed by hospitals. The National Safety Council (NSC) reports that hospital employees are 41% more likely to need time off due to injury or illness than employees in other industries. A survey of 165 clinical laboratories in Minnesota showed that the most frequent type of injuries were needle sticks (63%) followed by cuts and scrapes (21%). Hospital workers frequently report stress as a predisposing factor for accidents. Sprains and strains (often representing low back injury) were the most common type of workers compensation claim in 1983 as reported by the Bureau of Labor Statistics.

Guidance

In 1988, NIOSH published *Guidelines for Protecting the Safety and Health of Health Care Workers*; the American Association of Critical-Care Nurses has published a handbook on the occupational hazards encountered in the critical care environment; and the NSC has a Safety Guide for hospital environments. The hazards of exposure to waste, anesthetic gases, cytotoxic drugs, and blood-borne diseases such as hepatitis and HIV/AIDS are the subject of NIOSH criteria documents and OSHA policy statements.

Typical Hazards and Health Effects

This chapter covers hospital or health care facility-specific employee hazards. Biological, chemical and physical agents presenting potential exposure to health care employees are reviewed in Appendices VI:1-1 through VI:1-3. These lists are not inclusive.

Investigation Guidelines

Hospital Records

Hospital's OSHA 200 Log versus employee medical clinic care of employees-is there a possible trend in injuries and illnesses related to typical hazards? If available, check the hospital's safety program records and facility-enabling or operation equipment licenses, e.g., NRC radioisotope and radiation-source license.

Hospital Safety Programme

Note any previous health and safety inspections by local health departments, fire departments, regulatory or accrediting agencies, such as the Joint Commission on Accreditation of Healthcare Organisations (JCAHO), College of American Pathologists (CAP), and the American Osteopathic Association (AOA).

The policies and procedures should outline the training that all employees must receive. General hospital training should include fire and electrical safety, infection control procedures, and the hazard communication program. The policies and procedures should also delineate appropriate personnel and methods for preparation, mixing, application, storage, removal, and disposal of any hazardous agents. Emergency procedures should include provisions for fires, chemical or radioactive spills, extensive blood or body fluid spills, release of compressed, toxic, and corrosive gases, and power failure. A safety committee and/or infection control committee should be established within the hospital. Periodic inspection and monitoring is the responsibility of the safety committee. Immunisations, other than the mandatory vaccination for Hepatitis B, should be offered to personnel at risk.

All electrical equipment used in the hospital must be approved for safety by Underwriters Laboratory (UL) or another OSHA-approved body. Biosafety cabinets should be labeled and certified by the manufacturer and/or a safety officer. The cabinets should be placed in the room at a position where doors, windows, and traffic flow will not create turbulence around the face of the cabinet.

Walkround: Informal Interviews

The worker interviews should concentrate on compliance with appropriate policies and procedures. The employee should be able to verbalize what actions to take in the event of an emergency, i.e., accidental chemical or radioactive spill.

The employee should be aware of the hazards of the products with which he or she works. Observe the employees' lifting practices. Observe the Walkaround Inspection for Health Hazards.

Screening Samples

All sampling is based on the CSHO's professional judgment.

1. Sampling Methods.
2. When sampling, it is important to ensure that it is a typical day, i.e. normal exposure time.

3. Bioaerosols can be evaluated using the ACGIH Bioaerosol Committee's Guidelines. These guidelines contain information on sampling, analysis, and recommendations for remedial actions. Hospital infection control personnel should assist in bioaerosol determinations, as this is nonroutine sampling and is specific for preidentified organisms. Specialized bioaerosol sampling equipment is available through the OSHA Health Response Team.
4. Some of the most commonly found chemicals, e.g., formaldehyde, xylene, halothane, and acrylamide, can be screened using detector tubes. For nitrous oxide, passive monitors can be used to monitor exposure as stated in OSHA Method No. ID-166. Specific sampling for chemical agents, such as ethylene oxide, methyl methacrylate, ribavirin, nitrous oxide, halothane, and other waste anesthetic gases, can be found in the Chemical Information Manual.
5. Lasers are calibrated by the manufacturer, but the laser system must be checked prior to each procedure and during extended procedures. Classifications of lasers must coincide with actual measurement of output . Generally, measurements are required when the manufacturer's information is not available, when the laser system has not been classified or when alterations have been made to the laser system that may have changed its classification. Measurements should only be made by personnel trained in laser technology.
6. With regard to X-ray machines, film badges or their equivalent should be used for long-term monitoring. Ionizing radiation (x-ray)-Screening of radiation levels may be performed by using

thermoluminescence detectors, pocket dosimeters, and Geiger-Mueller counters.

7. Electrical equipment used in the hospital must follow Hospital Grades under Underwriter's Laboratory (UL) Standards 498 and 544. Resistance measurement and leakage measurements can be determined using the criteria in the National Fire Protection Association's *Health Care Facilities Handbook*.

Laser Classifications

Class 1	The least-hazardous class. Considered incapable of providing damaging levels of laser emissions.
Class 2	Applies only to visible laser emissions and may be viewed directly for time periods of less than or equal to 0.25 seconds, which is the aversion response time.
Class 3a	Dangerous under direct or reflected vision. These lasers are restricted to the visible electromagnetic spectrum.
Class 3b	May extend across the whole electromagnetic spectrum and are hazardous when viewed intrabeam.
Class 4	The highest-energy class of lasers, also extending across the electromagnetic spectrum. This class of laser presents significant fire, skin, and eye hazards.

Controls and Preventions

Engineering

All rooms should have adequate ventilation to remove contaminants. If air recirculation is required, then adequate filtering must be installed.

Intensive care units (ICU's), particularly neonatal ICU's, may be designed without walls between patient spaces. This may allow aerosolized chemicals and x-ray radiation to escape to neighboring areas.

Local Ventilation

General Points

a. Hoods should be used for specific procedures, such as mixing antineoplastic drugs. A scavenging system that contains a proper gas disposal system must be in place and operable.

b. Portable suction devices may be used for direct removal of contaminants. Portable ventilation should be used for smoke plume removal during laser surgery.

c. Ethylene oxide should be ventilated through a nonrecycled or dedicated ventilation system. For a discussion of ventilation of aeration units, sterilizer door areas, sterilizer relief valves, and ventilation during cylinder changes, see the appendix of 29 CFR 1910.1047 (Ethylene Oxide). Alarms for inadequate ventilation and automatic shutdown should be in place. Air pressure in laboratories and isolation rooms should be negative so that contaminated air is drawn through the exhaust vents rather than circulating throughout the rest of the building.

d. Biological safety cabinets are primary containment devices used by workers when handling moderate and high risk organisms. There are three types of biological safety cabinets:

— Class I: Open fronted, negative pressure, ventilated cabinet.

— Class II: HEPA-filtered, recirculated air cabinet with an open front face.

— Class III: A totally enclosed HEPA-filtered cabinet of gas-tight construction.

A class-III biological safety cabinet provides the highest protection to a worker. The effectiveness of the biological safety cabinets is dependent on air flow; therefore, the front intake grill and rear exhaust grill should not be blocked.

e. All windows must be covered or blacked out in laser surgical areas for protection of employees outside the surgical area.

f. Installation of automatic fire and explosion detection and protection equipment is recommended. The type should be specific to the hazard in the area.

g. In the morgue, local vacuum systems should be in place for power saws. Shields should be in place when significant splash hazards are anticipated.

h. There should be a separate storage area for radioactive sources. This area should be adequately shielded.

i. Laser systems, especially ones with high voltage capacitance, should be adequately covered. Also, bleeders and proper grounding should be attached to the system. All operating room doors to rooms that house lasers should contain safety interlocks, which shutdown the laser system if anyone enters the room.

j. Mixing of Methyl Methacrylate should be done in a closed system.

k. Ultraviolet lamps have been used to prevent tuberculosis transmission.

Administrative

a. Workers should receive health and safety training.
b. Vaccination for rubella, measles, mumps, and influenza is recommended, especially for women of child-bearing age.
c. Work-related stressors, such as inadequate work space, unreasonable work load, lack of readily available resources, inadequate and unsafe equipment, should be considered.
d. Appropriate emergency equipment (i.e., fire extinguishers, showers, eye wash) should be readily available.
e. Perform periodic environmental sampling when indicated.
f. Replace hazardous substances with less hazardous substances whenever possible (i.e., plastic for glass, small packets of chemicals, pre-poured formalin containers). Provide appropriate containers for disposal of sharps, hazardous waste, personal protective equipment.
g. Provide conveniently located and supplied hand washing facilities.
h. Document and retain inventories of radioactive materials. Only authorized personnel should have access to storage areas.

Maintenance Schedules

a. Hospital-grade electrical equipment including anesthesia machines, portable x-ray machines and laser systems, biological safety cabinets, and exhaust ventilation systems should have a preventive maintenance schedule. Testing intervals of electric equipment shall be set by the institution.

b. A specific person should have the responsibility for assuring proper maintenance of the portable x-ray machines. Preventive and corrective maintenance programs for x-ray machines are detailed in 21 CFR 1000, Radiological Health.

c. The anesthesia machine should be inspected and maintained at least every four months. This should be done by factory service representatives or other qualified personnel. Leakage of gas should be less than 100 ml/min during normal operation.

d. The entire laser system should be properly maintained and serviced according to the manufacturer's instructions. Only qualified personnel from the manufacturer or in-house shall maintain the system. Maintenance may only be done according to written standard operating procedures.

e. A written log is recommended for any detected leak and any service done on an ethylene oxide chamber. Sterilizer/aerator door gaskets, valves, and fittings must be replaced when necessary.

Training

a. All hospital staff members should have training on electrical and fire safety, hazard communication, and infection control by qualified personnel. Some educators recommend hands on training with pre- and post-tests.

b. In the hospital, specific training regarding hazardous substances should be given. Only qualified personnel may handle the hazardous substances or operate the specified machines.

Warning Signs

a. Specific requirements regarding the warning signs

to be used on electrical equipment are outlined in UL No. 544. This should include a Hospital Grade warning. Warning signs should be placed in areas where exposure to ribavirin, antineoplastic agent spills, ethylene oxide, or lasers is likely to occur.

b. Contract employees should not endanger hospital employees and can be controlled sometimes through use of privileges contracts.

Work Practices

Hands should be washed frequently and thoroughly. Workers should wash immediately after direct contact with any chemical, drug, blood, or other body fluid.

No eating, drinking, smoking or application of cosmetics should take place in the lab.

Needles and other sharp objects should be disposed of promptly in impervious containers. Needles should not be clipped or recapped by hand. See CPL 2-2.44B.

There should be immediate and proper disposal of biohazardous waste.

Mouth pipetting is to be prohibited.

Care should be taken not to create aerosols.

Appropriate personal dosimetry devices should be worn when working with radioactive materials.

Electrical equipment that appears to be damaged or in poor repair should not be used. Any shocks from electrical equipment should be reported promptly to the maintenance department.

Cylinders of compressed gases should be kept secured. They should never be dropped or allowed to strike each other with force.

Large pieces of broken glass should be removed with brooms and disposed of in a separate container. Small pieces can be removed with tongs. Glass should never be removed with fingers.

Vaporizers of anesthesia machines should be turned off when not in use. Also, proper face masks, sufficiently inflated endotracheal tubes, and prevention of anesthetic spills will decrease the amount of waste anesthetic gases in the operating room.

Antineoplastic drug contact requires the use of an isotonic wash to the body or eyes.

Personal Protective Equipment

Lab coats should be worn in the laboratory area and removed before leaving. Plastic or rubber aprons should be worn when there is a potential for splashing. Gloves should be worn when performing tasks such as handling hazardous chemicals, specimens, or hot materials. The type of glove should be selected according to the task being performed, as follows:

- Latex or vinyl type gloves should be changed frequently and inspected for punctures before putting them on.
- Double gloving to decrease the risk of exposure by penetration is recommended if it does not interfere with the task.
- Less permeable surgical latex gloves are recommended over polyvinyl gloves.
- Lead-lined gloves are to be worn in the direct x-ray field.

Rubber-soled shoes should be worn to prevent slips and falls. Rubber-lined shoe coverings may also be used to protect against spills or dropped objects. Fluid-proof shoes must be worn if there is a possibility of leakage to the skin.

Protective eyewear or shields should be used if splashes of a hazardous substance are likely to occur. Goggles that are tight-fitting may prevent irritation of the eyes if aerosolized chemicals are present. Goggles that protect the cornea, conjunctive and other ocular tissue are required for all personnel in the operating room during laser surgery. The wavelength of the laser output is the most important factor in determining the type of eye protection to be used. Opaque goggles are to be worn if in the direct x-ray field. Impervious or low permeability gowns should be worn when in contact with antineoplastic drugs, ribavirin and blood/ body fluids. These gowns should be properly stored in the area of use if contaminated. Soiled gowns should be washed or discarded. Lead-lined aprons are to be worn if in the x-ray field. Respirators may be required in case of emergencies, such as accidental spills and/or exposure to specific chemicals, e.g., formaldehyde and ethylene oxide. Check for a respirator program.

IMPACT OF BARRIER PRECAUTIONS IN REDUCING THE TRANSMISSION OF SERIOUS NOSOCOMIAL INFECTIONS

Many nosocomial infections are easily transferable from patient-to-patient, either via the hands of healthcare workers, or through the contamination of inanimate objects, including clothing and equipment. For some infections, the threat to other patients is considered serious enough that many institutions employ special barrier precautions, such as the use of gloves, gowns and disposable equipment for all patient contact, in caring for patients colonized or infected with these pathogens. Vancomycin-resistant enterococci (VRE) and *Clostridium difficile* represent 2 typical examples of nosocomial pathogens that may trigger such precautions. Although adherence to barrier precautions to prevent the spread of particularly concerning nosocomial pathogens has obvious face validity, the utility of specific interventions and the optimal forms they should take remain unclear. This uncertainty may in part reflect the impact of particular aspects of the epidemiology of the targeted nosocomial pathogens—i.e., the benefit of a given strategy may vary in different settings and with different organisms. Consequently, this chapter contrasts with the review of handwashing, a practice for which the benefit was regarded as sufficiently established to warrant focusing on strategies for improving compliance. While compliance with barrier precautions is also an important topic and likely plays a significant role in the efficacy of such interventions, this chapter analyses the literature evaluating the benefit of the barrier precautions themselves.

Prevalence and Severity of the Target Safety Problem

Nosocomial infections, including *C. difficile*-associated diarrhea and VRE, significantly increase the morbidity and mortality of hospitalized patients. Both infections are also associated with increased hospital costs. Recent evidence also suggests there may be a relationship between *C. difficile* and VRE, with *C. difficile* infection identified as a risk factor for VRE infection. The increased incidence of both VRE and *C. difficile* can be attributed to spread from patient to patient. Failure to recognize these dissemination patterns may result in an inability to contain outbreaks when they occur in the hospital.

C. difficile has been identified as the major, if not only, important cause of infectious diarrhea that develops in patients after hospitalisation, occurring in up to 30% of adult hospitalized patients who developed diarrhea. One study found an acquisition rate of 13% for patients hospitalized 1-2 weeks, which increased to 50% for patients hospitalized >4 weeks. In addition, the incidence of *C. difficile* infection has increased in recent years, with one study reporting a 5-fold increase in clinical infection between 1993 and 1996. *C. difficile* infection increases lengths of stay, often to as long as 18-30 days and, when fulminant, can lead to exploratory and therapeutic surgical procedures. Mortality attributable to *C. difficile*, while reported, occurs in fewer than 5% of patients. The costs associated with *C. difficile* diarrhea, while not well described, may be as high as $10,000 per patient.

VRE, first described in 1988, currently accounts for greater than 25% of all nosocomial enterococci. Early national data suggested that infections with VRE were associated with mortality rates of over 36%, more than double that of patients with vancomycin-susceptible (VSE) infections. While later studies called some of these results into question, the most recent studies have again suggested that vancomycin-resistance carries an independent effect on mortality. VRE infections are also associated with significantly higher hospital costs than those due to VSE.

Although *C. difficile* and VRE are among the most common nosocomial pathogens that have significant effects on morbidity, mortality, and cost, there are a number of other nosocomial pathogens which could also be studied. These include pathogens such as methicillin-resistant *Staphylococcus aureus* (MRSA), extended-spectrum beta-lactamase (ESBL) producing *Enterobacteriaceae*, *Acinetobacter* species, and *Pseudomonas aeruginosa*. While these are all important nosocomial pathogens, *C. difficile* and VRE were chosen as examples because they are extremely common, and they represent both antibiotic-susceptible (*C. difficile*) and antibiotic-resistant (VRE) pathogens.

Additionally, (unlike MRSA and *P. aeruginosa*) the epidemiology of both pathogens is complex, representing both person-to-person spread and association with prior antibiotic use, allowing for a more comprehensive discussion of the relative merits of both antimicrobial use interventions and barrier precaution interventions.

Practice Description

Barrier precautions include any activity designed to prevent the spread of nosocomial pathogens from patient to patient. This chapter reviews the following 3 practices:

— *Use of gowns and gloves for all contact with patients colonized or infected with VRE and/or C. difficile*: Healthcare workers typically don gloves and gowns when entering the room of an infected or colonized patient, and remove them upon exiting (followed immediately by handwashing) to reduce the likelihood of clothing or equipment contamination that could transmit pathogens to other patients.

— *Use of dedicated or disposable examining equipment for patients colonized or infected with VRE and/or C. difficile*: Hospital equipment (i.e., blood pressure cuffs, thermometers) remains in a patient's room and is not carried from room to room.

— *Patient and/or staff cohorting for patients colonized or infected with VRE and/or C. difficile*: Patients colonized or infected with similar pathogens are admitted to specific floors of the hospital where designated healthcare workers care only for patients colonized or infected with these pathogens.

Study Designs

A structured search of the PubMed database (including MEDLINE) and review of the bibliographies of relevant articles identified 19 studies that have examined the implementation of barrier precaution practices designed to impact the incidence of VRE and/or *C. difficile* infection. All studies found on literature search were included in this review except for those reporting very small outbreaks (defined as fewer than 10 cases of *C. difficile* or VRE). Sixteen of the reviewed studies were before-after observational cohort studies (Level 3), in which baseline data regarding incidence of VRE or *C. difficile* were obtained during an observational period and compared to a second period after implementation of an intervention. Crude comparability data on the before and after groups (e.g., total admissions, patient census) were provided in 2 reports while only one study statistically compared the before and after groups to assess comparability. Three reports detailed unblinded comparative studies (Level 2) in which patients on different wards were assigned different interventions. Each of these studies assessed the comparability of the study groups on the basis of underlying demographic variables.

Study Outcomes

All of the studies reviewed reported changes in the incidence or prevalence of either VRE or *C. difficile* as a result of barrier precaution interventions (Level 1). For studies investigating *C. difficile*, all outcomes were reported in terms of clinical infections. For studies investigating VRE, outcomes were reported as VRE colonisation and/or infection rates.

Opportunities for Impact

As noted above, both VRE and *C. difficile* affect a large proportion of hospitalized patients. Improvements in barrier precaution interventions against these pathogens would have a tremendous impact. There are few data regarding the percentage of hospitals that employ any one of a number of barrier precautions (e.g., gowns, gloves, disposable thermometers). In addition, while standard practice is to apply barrier precautions for patients with nosocomial pathogens with demonstrated horizontal spread, compliance with precautions is frequently poor, often below 50%. Purported reasons for this lack of compliance include lack of resources and busy staff workload. Regardless, these results suggest that the opportunity for improvement in these practices is great.

Evidence for Effectiveness of the Practice

As both VRE and *C. difficile* have clearly been shown to be transferable from patient-to-patient, interventions designed to improve barrier precautions yield significant reductions in the incidence of infection with these two pathogens. All studies that examined the effect of enhanced barrier precautions on *C. difficile* infection demonstrated benefit, suggesting that barrier precaution interventions are effective in controlling its emergence. Most studies employed a multifaceted approach including several different barrier precaution components. For example, one study combined use of vinyl gloves and ongoing educational interventions, another included cohorting, culture screening, and daily room disinfection, while another combined reinforcement of enteric precautions, replacement of electronic thermometers, and institution of closed paper towel dispensers. Given the varied components of barrier precaution interventions instituted in different studies, it is difficult to determine the specific effect of any individual component.

The evidence of effectiveness of barrier precautions for VRE is somewhat less clear-cut. All but 4 of the studies examining the effect of barrier precautions on VRE demonstrated a benefit, but study design differences and particular epidemiologic trends may account for the inconsistent findings.

One of the 4 studies that noted no significant effect compared glove use to glove and gown use. The second noted that the emergence of VRE at the study institution was due to multiple genetically-unrelated strains, suggesting that person-to-person spread was less important at that site. It is thus not surprising that barrier precautions would have less of an effect. In the third study, routine rectal swab surveillance and contact precautions were instituted in response to a clinical outbreak of VRE and surveillance was continued for only 6 months. Since surveillance was not conducted prior to institution of precautions, it is impossible to say what the colonisation prevalence had been prior to the intervention. Furthermore, as the authors point out, it may be that the outbreak would have been much worse had the precautions not been put in place. Finally, no determination of genetic relatedness (and hence spread) was made in this study. In the fourth study, while there was a reduction in the isolation of VRE, there was not complete eradication. According to the authors, the most likely reason for this less-than-optimal response was poor compliance with contact precaution guidelines.

Thus, it appears that enhanced barrier precautions are generally effective in reducing the incidence of VRE but that various aspects of both the epidemiology of the VRE outbreak and the implementation of guidelines may temper the effectiveness of interventions. Similar to the studies investigating response of *C. difficile* to barrier precautions, most studies of VRE employed several components of barrier precautions as part of a multifaceted approach. It is thus difficult to determine the specific effect of any individual component.

Potential for Harm

None of the reviewed studies reported any assessment of possible harm as a result of the barrier precaution interventions. In fact, the implementation of barrier precautions is unlikely to result in harm to the patient. One potential concern is that time necessary to comply with the interventions (e.g., gowning, gloving), might make healthcare workers less likely to complete tasks necessary to provide acceptable patient care. Indeed, it has recently been noted that healthcare workers were half as likely to enter the rooms of patients on contact isolation. Furthermore, while contact precautions appeared to have little effect on patient examination by resident physicians, attending physicians were 50% less likely to examine a patient on contact precautions compared to a patient not on precautions. Future studies should address these concerns by documenting the time required to adhere to barrier precautions, and determining the potential impact of precautions on patient care.

Another potentially harmful consequence of barrier precaution interventions is the psychological effect that contact precautions may have on the isolated patient. While research has examined the effects of sensory deprivation and social isolation, a recent review of the literature noted little progress in the investigation of the psychological effects of contact isolation.

Costs and Implementation

It seems apparent that the more complicated an intervention, the less likely healthcare workers will adhere to it. While 2 studies noted compliance with barrier precautions at close to 90%, others noted levels closer to 70%. One study actually noted compliance levels to be significantly higher in those healthcare workers who used both gowns and gloves compared to those using only gowns. This somewhat counterintuitive finding suggests that other factors may be at play in influencing compliance. Of the reviewed studies that reported compliance levels, all did so relatively shortly after the initial implementation of interventions. Future studies should assess compliance with guidelines over a longer period.

Four studies reported the costs of specific interventions. Implementation of use of disposable thermometers was estimated at $14,055 per year at a 343-bed institution. Another study of the impact of disposable thermometers estimated that the cost per prevented *C. difficile* infection would be approximately $611. A study using a multifaceted approach estimated that the annual expenses due directly to increased demand for gowns and gloves were approximately $11,000. Finally, a multifaceted intervention at a 254-bed long-term care facility which included education, gowns and gloves for resident contact, no sharing of personal equipment, and daily double cleaning of resident rooms and wheelchairs, estimated the total cost of the intervention to be $12,061 Canadian (approximately $8000 US).

The costs of implementing a program to enhance barrier precaution practices must be balanced against the potential cost savings due to decreased incidence of nosocomial infections. Both VRE and *C. difficile* infections have been associated with significantly increased length of hospital stay. Preventing even a small number of these infections is likely to have a significant financial impact. While several of the reviewed studies documented costs associated with various interventions, no study systematically compared these costs to the potential cost savings of infections prevented.

Comment

The majority of reviewed studies demonstrated a significant reduction in the incidence of VRE or *C. difficile* following barrier precaution interventions. The fact that not all studies found a benefit suggests that future studies should identify those scenarios (e.g., outbreak, endemic colonisation, etc.) in which attention to barrier precautions is most likely to be beneficial. In addition, it is possible that a combined intervention involving both enhanced barrier precautions as well as antibiotic formulary interventions might be needed in order to effect the greatest possible change in VRE and *C. difficile* infection rates. While these studies, much like those that examined the impact of antibiotic use practices, demonstrated short-term success, future studies should determine the efficacy of such interventions over the long term. Finally, the cost-effectiveness of such strategies should be investigated.

IMPACT OF CHANGES IN ANTIBIOTIC USE PRACTICES ON NOSOCOMIAL INFECTIONS AND ANTIMICROBIAL RESISTANCE—*CLOSTRIDIUM DIFFICILE* AND VANCOMYCIN-RESISTANT ENTEROCOCCUS (VRE)

As discussed in the chapters on handwashing and barrier precautions, hospital infection control has historically focused on preventing the transmission of nosocomial pathogens—either from patient to patient or from provider to patient. The potential role of overseeing hospital-wide antibiotic use as an infection control measure has also been recognized for many years. With the widespread emergence of nosocomial antibiotic-resistant infections over the past 10-15 years, institutional efforts to control antibiotic use have become a priority for infection control.

The practices reviewed in this chapter involve institutional efforts to control antibiotic use as a means of controlling complications of antibiotic overuse or misuse.

In evaluating the potential benefits of these practices, the focus is on the impacts of antibiotic use on infections with vancomycin-resistant enterococci (VRE) and *Clostridium difficile*. These pathogens represent two of the most important nosocomial pathogens with relationships to inappropriate antibiotic use. Moreover, as suggested by recent evidence, infection with *C. difficile* may represent a risk factor for infection with VRE.

Practice Description

Interventions designed to limit the use of antibiotics may take many forms. Specific practices reviewed in the chapter include:

— *Infectious diseases physician approval*—all requests for an antibiotic are discussed with an infectious diseases physician who decides whether use is appropriate.

— *Monitoring of antibiotic use by pharmacy service*—pharmacists monitor the use of certain antibiotics and make recommendations for changes to the prescriber.

— *Guidelines for antimicrobial use*—dissemination to physicians of guidelines describing appropriate and inappropriate use.

— *Therapeutic substitution*—use of one agent replaced by another agent with similar spectrum of activity.

— *Computer-assisted prescribing*—computer-based restriction of agent with extra prompts requesting documentation of indication for agent.

— *Antibiotic-management program (AMP)*—continuation of antibiotic after a specific duration requires approval from either an infectious diseases physician or pharmacist on the AMP.

Prevalence and Severity of the Target Safety Problem

This study focuses 2 of the most important nosocomial pathogens: VRE and *C. difficile*. VRE currently accounts for greater than 25% of all nosocomial enterococci and confers an increased risk of death, independent of comorbid conditions that may have initially led to the infection. VRE infections are also associated with significantly higher hospital costs than those due to vancomycin-sensitive enterococci (VSE). *C. difficile* represents the major, if not only, important infectious cause of nosocomial diarrhea. Although death attributable to *C. difficile* occurs in less than 5% of patients, the impact of *C. difficile* infection remains significant. Patients may require substantially longer lengths of hospital stay—upwards of 18-30 days, with exploratory and therapeutic surgical procedures required in severe cases. It has also been suggested that more debilitated patients (e.g., in rehabilitation centers or long-term care facilities) may be at even greater risk for increased morbidity and mortality due to *C. difficile* infection. The costs associated with *C. difficile* diarrhea, while not well described, are estimated to be as high as $10,000 per patient.

Opportunities for Impact

Over half of all hospitalized patients are treated with antibiotics. The antibiotics represent a significant portion of overall healthcare costs, accounting for between 20% and 50% of total hospital drug expenditures. It has been estimated that 50% of all antibiotics prescribed are either at the wrong dose, the wrong drug, or taken for the wrong duration. These findings suggest that there is significant room for improvement in antibiotic prescribing practices. Most hospitals employ formulary restrictions for certain medications (particularly expensive agents, selecting one drug from a group of equivalent agents). However, only a minority of hospitals uses formulary restrictions to limit the use of entire antibiotic classes or specific agents. Those hospitals that do employ antimicrobial formulary restrictions most often do so as a means of controlling costs, rather than as an infection control measure. Thus, there remain substantial opportunities to expand upon these existing formulary programs to control the emergence of antimicrobial resistance.

Study Designs

A structured search of the PubMed database (including MEDLINE) and review of the bibliographies of relevant articles identified 10 studies that have examined methods to change antibiotic use with respect to VRE and/or *C. difficile* infection. All of these studies were before-after observational cohort studies (Level 3) in which baseline data regarding incidence of VRE or *C. difficile* were obtained during an observational period and compared with a second time period after an intervention had been implemented. Data on baseline comparability of the before and after groups were not reported in 6 studies. Two studies only reported similar admission and census rates during the before and after time periods, while 2 studies compared patients in the 2 time periods on the basis of numerous variables.

Study Outcomes

All of the studies reviewed reported changes in the clinical incidence or prevalence of either VRE or *C. difficile* as a result of antibiotic practice interventions. Studies investigating *C. difficile* measured clinical infections. Studies investigating VRE examined VRE infection or VRE colonisation.

Evidence for Effectiveness of the Practice

Several possibilities may explain the negative findings of these 3 studies. First, the interventions analysed might not have produced significant alterations in antibiotic use, so that infection rates with the target pathogens remained unchanged. Second, it is possible that patient-to-patient spread of these pathogens limited the efficacy of the interventions, as this mode of transmission is well known to occur for both VRE and *C. difficile*, usually via the hands of healthcare workers. Third, since environmental contamination occurs with both these pathogens, successful control of these organisms may require enhanced disinfection procedures in scme cases. Targeting antibiotic use may not be sufficient to reduce incidence of these pathogens since a significant number of infected or colonized patients may serve as reservoirs. Under this scenario, the argument for barrier precautions as an adjunct measure to prevent spread of organisms from patient to patient becomes more persuasive. Indeed, although changes in antibiotic use practice were the primary intervention in all of the studies reviewed here, one study included a component of enhanced barrier precautions in the intervention. Future studies should investigate the impact of such multifaceted interventions, both for VRE and *C. difficile* as well as for other nosocomial pathogens.

Other Potential Benefits

Although not the focus of this , the practices reviewed here may have a beneficial impact on other emerging nosocomial pathogens strongly associated with inappropriate antibiotic use, such as extended-spectrum beta-lactamase (ESBL) producing *Enterobacteriaceae*. In addition, although we have focused on control of VRE as an end in itself, a primary motivation to achieve this goal is the need to delay the emergence of vancomycin-resistance in *Staphylococcus aureus*. As *S. aureus* represents the most common nosocomial infection, the development of high-level vancomycin resistance among staphylococci would constitute a public health disaster.

Thus, practices that decrease the prevalence of VRE may play an important, albeit indirect, role in preventing or delaying this occurrence.

Potential for Harm

Few of the reviewed studies reported any assessment of possible harm as a result of the antibiotic use practice interventions. One potential result of interventions designed to reduce the use of one antibiotic, or antibiotic class, is the subsequent increase in the use of another class of agents to compensate. In fact, one reviewed study noted an increase in the use of other anti-anaerobic agents as clindamycin use decreased. Whether changes in antibiotic use results in changes in antimicrobial susceptibilities, either in the pathogen under study (e.g., VRE, *C. difficile*) or in other nosocomial pathogens, it is a fertile ground for future study. Finally, efforts to decrease use of certain antibiotics might increase infection rates due to inappropriate withholding of appropriate antibiotics. However, one reviewed study noted no increase in rates of surgical site infections following decrease in the use of vancomycin for preoperative prophylaxis.

Costs and Implementation

The costs of implementing a program to alter antibiotic use practices must be balanced against potential cost savings. Sources of savings may be reduced antibiotic use, use of less expensive agents rather than the more expensive newer agents, and potentially, reduced costs due to decreased incidence of nosocomial infections as a result of interventions. Although several studies reported cost savings due only to decreased antibiotic use, analyses taking into account costs related to subsequent infections (or infections prevented) have been sparse. One study noted that cost savings from decreased use of clindamycin offset the expenditures due to increased use of other antibiotics. The authors suggested that if each case of *C. difficile* resulted in a cost of $2000, the savings to the hospital of the intervention could approach $162,000 annually based on the number of cases averted.

Another cost of antibiotic use interventions is the expense of ongoing monitoring of antibiotic use and antimicrobial susceptibilities of nosocomial pathogens. Effective recommendation of certain antimicrobial agents over others requires access to (and financial and logistic support for) routine antimicrobial susceptibility testing. Monitoring institutional resistance patterns is vital in order to make required formulary changes in response to emerging resistance patterns and to determine the most effective agents given prevailing susceptibility patterns.

Comment

Given the strong association between antibiotic use and subsequent infection (demonstrated for both *C. difficile* and VRE), it is not surprising that changes in antibiotic use practices can reduce the incidence of infection with these 2 pathogens. The majority of reviewed studies demonstrated a significant reduction in the incidence of VRE or *C. difficile* following interventions to change antibiotic use practice. While these studies all demonstrated short-term success, future studies should confirm the efficacy of such interventions over the long term. In addition, the effectiveness and feasibility of combining antibiotic practice strategies with efforts to enhance barrier precautions should be investigated. Finally, the cost-effectiveness of such strategies (taking into account both the costs associated with monitoring and maintaining sound antibiotic use practices and the costs associated with nosocomial antibiotic-resistant infections) should be investigated.

PREVENTION OF NOSOCOMIAL URINARY TRACT INFECTIONS

Many hospitalized patients require the placement of indwelling urinary catheters for days or even weeks at a time. Only a minority of patients develop urinary tract infections because of the presence of these devices, but the frequency of their use produces substantial overall morbidity for patients and costs to the healthcare system. Urinary tract infections (UTIs) account for up to 40% of nosocomial infections, with urinary catheter-related infections causing the vast majority of nosocomial UTIs. Each hospital-acquired UTI adds approximately $675 to the costs of hospitalisation. When bacteremia develops, this additional cost increases to at least $2800.

Because of the substantial complications and costs associated with the use of urinary catheters, a number of practices have been evaluated in an effort to reduce the incidence of urinary catheter-related infections. This chapter reviews the evidence supporting the use of silver alloy coated urinary catheters, and, because of its similarity, the recently described practice of using urinary catheters impregnated with the antibiotic combination of minocycline and rifampin.

Practice Description

Silver is a highly effective antibacterial substance, which can be applied to various types of catheters. Multiple studies have suggested that silicone urethral catheters coated with hydrogel and silver salts reduce the risk of developing bacteriuria, compared with standard latex urethral catheters (Foley catheters). As shown in a recent meta-analysis, this benefit applies to catheters coated with silver alloy (which are coated on both internal and external surfaces of the catheter), but not silver oxide (which are coated on the external catheter surface only). Consequently, this chapter focuses only on studies evaluating silver alloy catheters, and the use of catheters coated with antimicrobials.

Prevalence and Severity of the Target Safety Problem

Almost one million episodes of nosocomial UTI occur annually in the United States. Each year approximately 96 million urethral catheters are sold worldwide. Of these, nearly 25% are sold in the United States. The daily rate of bacteriuria in catheterized patients ranges from 3 to 10%, with the incidence directly related to the duration of catheterisation. Among patients with bacteriuria, 10 to 25% will develop symptoms of local urinary tract infection, such as suprapubic or flank pain. The development of catheter-related bacteriuria carries with it a 2.8-fold increased risk of death, independent of other co-morbid conditions and disease severity. Bacteremia results from catheter-related bacteriuria in approximately 3% of patients, and invariably represents a serious complication.

Beyond the morbidity and mortality associated with indwelling catheters, catheter-related infection results in substantially increased healthcare costs. Data suggest that each episode of hospital-acquired symptomatic catheter-related UTI costs an additional $676, and each episode of catheter-related nosocomial bacteremia costs a minimum of $2836. Estimates from one university hospital, based on data from almost 20 years ago, were that hospital-acquired UTI led to approximately $204,000 in additional expenses per year. More recent data are unavailable, but the institutional costs attributable to catheter-related infection are clearly substantial.

Opportunities for Impact

Since catheter-related UTI is the leading cause of nosocomial infection in the United States and is associated with increased morbidity and costs, any intervention that reduces the incidence of catheter-related UTI is potentially important. Currently, it is unknown what proportion of patients with indwelling catheters receives silver alloy catheters, however it is likely to be the minority.

Study Designs

A meta-analysis which included 4 randomized clinical trials, compared the efficacy of silver catheters with standard, non-coated catheters. Five additional studies have appeared since publication of this meta-analysis. In 3 of these studies, the patient represented the unit of analysis. Another study employed a randomized crossover design (Level 1), randomizing wards rather than individual patients. The final study used a prospective, before-after design at 5 different hospitals (Level 2).

The patient populations for these studies included patients on various hospital services including urology, internal medicine, neurology, and the intensive care unit. In general, the studies included patients expected to be catheterized for at least 2 days. Since the patients resided in acute care hospitals rather than extended care centers, most were catheterized for 10 days or less. Several studies specified that patients given concomitant antibiotics were excluded.

Study Outcomes

The individual trials and the meta-analysis focused primarily on the surrogate outcome of bacteriuria (Level 2). The definition of bacteriuria varied somewhat in the studies. However, low-level growth from a catheterized specimen (i.e., 10 colony forming units (CFU) /mL) usually progresses within days to concentrations of greater than 10 CFU/mL unless antibiotic therapy is given. Unfortunately, none of the studies was adequately powered to detect a significant difference in the clinically more important outcomes of catheter-related bacteremia or death. Though bacteriuria is a surrogate endpoint, it is probably appropriate to use since it is a component of the only causal pathway in the disease process between catheterisation and an important clinical outcome (e.g., symptomatic UTI or catheter-related bacteremia). One study did report differences in secondary bloodstream infections.

Evidence for Effectiveness of the Practice

The 4 clinical trials of silver alloy catheters included in the meta-analysis all showed a significant reduction in the development of catheter-associated bacteriuria. The meta-analysis have reported more mixed results. Several of the studies have shown a statistically significant benefit of silver alloy catheters, but with a smaller relative risk reduction compared to that reported in the meta-analysis. However, one study failed to find a significant benefit associated with silver alloy catheters, and another found benefit from silver alloy catheters in those given such catheters for about 5 days, but not in those given the catheter for 14 days. A formal update of the previous meta-analysis would be helpful, but is beyond the scope of the current report.

Potential for Harm

There is likely minimal harm from the use of silver alloy urinary catheters. The one theoretical harm involves the development of antimicrobial resistance. However, since silver is not used systemically in the form of an antimicrobial agent for treatment, the clinical significance of antimicrobial resistance to silver is unclear.

Costs and Implementation

Each silver alloy urinary catheter tray costs about $5.30 more than a standard, non-coated urinary catheter tray.

However, a recent economic evaluation indicates that when all the clinical and economic costs are accounted for, silver alloy urinary catheters may provide both clinical and economic benefits in patients receiving indwelling catheterisation for 2 to 10 days. It should be noted that one of the major assumptions made in the economic evaluation is that a certain proportion of patients with bacteriuria develop the clinically important (Level 1) outcomes of symptomatic UTI or bacteremia. The economic analysis did not assign any costs to bacteriuria but did assign costs if patients developed these clinically important outcomes. Additionally, several of the very recent efficacy studies of silver alloy catheters were not included in the economic analysis. A clinical study, adequately powered to detect both meaningful clinical and economic endpoints, would confirm the results of this economic evaluation that relied on modeling techniques. The overall cost of universal implementation of silver alloy catheters is unclear.

Comment

The data supporting the use of silver alloy urinary catheters to reduce urinary catheter-related bacteriuria is reasonably strong. As noted, the incidence of bacteriuria, while not extremely high, carries a high morbidity. It remains unclear whether silver alloy urinary catheters will also lead to decreases in the clinically more important outcomes of catheter-related bacteremia and mortality. Continuing investigation into the impact of silver alloy catheters on these important outcomes and their effect on the emergence of antibiotic resistance should be pursued. Of note, catheters coated with antibacterial substances other than silver have also been evaluated. A recent randomized study found that patients who received antimicrobial-impregnated catheters coated with minocycline and rifampin had significantly lower rates of gram-positive bacteriuria than a control group given standard, non-coated catheters (7.1% vs. 38.2%; $p < 0.001$). Both control and intervention groups had similar rates of gram-negative bacteriuria and candiduria. However, the theoretical risk of developing antimicrobial resistance to minocycline and/or rifampin (2 agents occasionally used systemically) may limit the use of catheters coated with these antibiotics.

PREVENTION OF VENTILATOR-ASSOCIATED PNEUMONIA

Ventilator-associated pneumonia (VAP) is a leading cause of morbidity and mortality in the intensive care unit (ICU). The incidence of VAP varies greatly, ranging from 6 to 52% of intubated patients depending on patient risk factors. The cumulative incidence is approximately 1-3% per day of intubation. Overall, VAP is associated with an attributable mortality of up to 30%. Attributable mortality approaches 50% when VAP is caused by the more virulent organisms that typify late-onset VAP (occurring 4 or more days into mechanical ventilation). The cost per episode of VAP is substantial, although specific data are lacking. The average cost per episode of nosocomial pneumonia is estimated at $3000 to $6000, and the additional length of stay for patients who develop VAP is estimated at 13 days.

VAP is typically categorized as either early-onset VAP (occurring in the first 3-4 days of mechanical ventilation) or late-onset VAP. This distinction is important microbiologically. Early-onset VAP is commonly caused by antibiotic-sensitive community-acquired organisms (e.g., *Streptococcus pneumoniae*, *Haemophilus influenzae*, and *Staphylococcus aureus*). Late-onset VAP is commonly caused by antibiotic-resistant nosocomial organisms (e.g., *Pseudomonas aeruginosa*, methicillin-resistant *Staphylococcus aureus*, *Acinetobacter* species, and

Enterobacter species). Most episodes of ventilator-associated pneumonia (VAP) are thought to develop from the aspiration of oropharyngeal secretions containing potentially pathogenic organisms. Aspiration of gastric secretions may also contribute, though likely to a lesser degree. Tracheal intubation interrupts the body's anatomic and physiologic defenses against aspiration, making mechanical ventilation a major risk factor for VAP.

This chapter reviews 4 practices that carry the potential to reduce the incidence of VAP in patients receiving mechanical ventilation. They are: variation in patient positioning, continuous aspiration of subglottic secretions, selective digestive tract decontamination, and the use of sucralfate. Aspiration of gastric secretions likely contributes to the development of VAP. Semi-recumbent positioning of mechanically ventilated patients may help reduce the incidence of gastroesophogeal reflux and lead to a decreased incidence of VAP. Immobility in critically ill patients leads to atelectasis and decreased clearance of bronchopulmonary secretions. Both of these sequelae may lead to increased risk of VAP. Continuous rotation and movement of critically ill patients (termed continuous oscillation) may thus help prevent such changes.

Semi-recumbent Positioning

Practice Description

Semi-recumbent positioning is generally defined as elevation of the head of the bed to 45 degrees. This is generally achieved in a hospital bed with patients' feet remaining parallel to the floor (i.e., the entire bed is not tilted) but this is not explicitly described in the published trials. Semi-recumbency is generally continued for the duration of mechanical ventilation.

Opportunities for Impact

Outside of select medical centers that have studied this practice, semi-recumbent positioning has not been widely adopted as the standard of care. Thus, such an intervention would have enormous opportunity for impact should it prove beneficial.

Study Designs

There have been three trials of semi-recumbent patient positioning and its effect on the incidence of VAP. Two of these studies measured aspiration events using nuclear medicine techniques, the other was a randomized trial with the primary outcome being VAP. In the one randomized trial, 86 patients were randomized at the time of intubation to semi-recumbent body position (45 degrees) or supine body position (0 degrees). All patients received the same general critical care (e.g., sterile endotracheal suctioning, stress ulcer prophylaxis with sucralfate if tolerating oral medications, no ventilator tubing changes, no selective digestive tract decontamination).

Study Outcomes

In the one randomized clinical trial, VAP was clinically defined as a new and persistent infiltrate on chest radiography, plus two of the following: temperature of >38.3C, leukocyte count >12,000/mm or <4000/mm, purulent tracheal secretions. Microbiologic confirmation required the above criteria be met and the isolation of pathogenic bacteria from an endotracheal aspirate or bronchoscopic procedure. Mortality was reported at time of discharge from the ICU. Both studies of the frequency of aspiration measured radioisotope counts (counts per minute) of endotracheal aspirates at various time points before during and after semi-recumbent positioning.

Potential for Harm

No adverse effects were observed in patients randomized to semi-recumbent positioning. However, patients were excluded if they had any of the following conditions: recent abdominal or neurologic surgery (<7 days), shock refractory to vasoactive therapy, and previous recent endotracheal intubation (<30 days).

Evidence for Effectiveness of the Practice

Only one randomized clinical trial of semi-recumbent patient positioning in mechanically ventilated patients has been published to date. Semi-recumbent positioning was associated with a statistically significant reduction in both clinically and microbiologically-diagnosed VAP. There was no significant difference in mortality. These findings corroborate earlier studies that demonstrated decreased frequency of gastroesophogeal reflux with semi-recumbent positioning, and an independent association of supine positioning with the development of VAP.

Costs and Implementation

The cost of semi-recumbent positioning is negligible and implementation is simple but will require healthcare provider education.

Continuous oscillation

Practice Description

Continuous oscillation utilizes mechanical beds that employ either rotating platforms or alternating inflation/deflation of mattress compartments to turn patients from side to side. These beds achieve 40 to 60 degrees of tilt and can cycle every 5-30 minutes as programmed. In general, in published trials, continuous oscillation was started within 24 hours of admission to the ICU and continued until discharge.

Opportunities for Impact

Continuous oscillation is infrequently applied to critically ill patients. Thus, this intervention would have significant opportunity for impact should it prove beneficial.

Study Designs

A meta-analysis of six randomized controlled trials evaluated the effect of continuous oscillation on clinical outcomes, including pneumonia, in critically ill patients. The vast majority of patients were mechanically ventilated but the absolute percentage is not reported in most trials. Five of the six trials included were limited to surgical and/or neurologic patients. A subsequent randomized controlled trial included 103 medical and surgical patients. In most cases, continuous oscillation was compared to standard critical care practice of rolling patients every two hours.

Study Outcomes

The definition of VAP varied among trials but was generally clinical and required a new infiltrate on chest radiography, fever, and leukocytosis. Microbiologic confirmation was not consistently obtained. Mortality was recorded at time of ICU discharge.

Evidence for Effectiveness of the Practice

The role of continuous oscillation in the prevention of VAP is unclear. A meta-analysis of six randomized controlled trials on this subject found a statistically significant reduction in the risk of pneumonia. Five of these studies were limited to surgical and/or neurologic patients. The sixth study, which included primarily medical patients, failed to find any significant effect. A subsequent randomized controlled trial of medical and surgical patients also failed to find any benefit.

Potential for Harm

There were no significant risks of continuous oscillation in any of the randomized trials. Inadvertent disconnection of intravenous lines, increased ventricular ectopy, and patient intolerance were reported, but not quantified. Conscious patients tolerated the procedure poorly.

Costs and Implementation

The incremental cost of specialized beds capable of continuous oscillation has been estimated at approximately $100 per day. A significant reduction in VAP incidence and length of stay could result in cost savings.

Comment

Both semi-recumbent positioning and continuous oscillation are relatively low-cost, low-risk interventions. The one randomized trial to date of semi-recumbent positioning shows it to be an effective method of reducing VAP. While it has not proven to provide a mortality benefit, semi-recumbent positioning is a safe and straightforward intervention whose effectiveness should be confirmed by additional randomized clinical trials. Continuous oscillation is less clearly beneficial, although it may be effective in certain subgroups of patients (e.g., surgical, neurologic). It also deserves continued study.

CONTINUOUS ASPIRATION OF SUBGLOTTIC SECRETIONS

Ventilator-associated pneumonia (VAP) frequently develops from the aspiration of oropharyngeal secretions containing potentially pathogenic organisms. Tracheal intubation interrupts the body's anatomic and physiologic defenses against aspiration, making mechanical ventilation a major risk factor for VAP. The accumulation of contaminated oropharyngeal secretions above the endotracheal tube cuff may contribute to the risk of aspiration. Removal of these pooled secretions through suctioning of the subglottic region, termed continuous aspiration of subglottic secretions (CASS), may reduce the risk of developing VAP.

Practice Description

Continuous aspiration of subglottic secretions requires intubation with specially designed endotracheal tubes. These endotracheal tubes contain a separate dorsal lumen that opens into the subglottic region, allowing for aspiration of any pooled secretions. The amount of secretions is monitored (usually daily) and the patency of the suction lumen is tested frequently (every few hours). In studies of the impact of this practice, aspiration has been applied from time of intubation to time of extubation. One of the studies tested manual aspiration performed hourly instead of continuous mechanical aspiration.

Opportunities for Impact

Continuous aspiration of subglottic secretions is an uncommon practice. The opportunities for impact are therefore significant should this practice prove beneficial in lowering rates of VAP.

Study Designs

There have been three randomized controlled trials of CASS to date. Two have included both medical and surgical patients requiring mechanical ventilation for greater than 72 hours and one included only post-cardiac surgery patients. All three studies randomized patients to CASS or standard care. Attempts were made to control for additional, potentially effective preventive strategies such as patient positioning, frequency of ventilator circuit changes, type of stress ulcer prophylaxis used, and administration of antibiotics.

Study Outcomes

All trials reported development of VAP and mortality at the time of extubation, ICU or hospital discharge. VAP was generally defined as a new radiographic infiltrate plus two of the following: fever, leukocytosis/leukopenia, or purulent tracheal aspirate. Microbiologic confirmation was not consistently obtained. Time to development of VAP was also reported. Mortality was reported at time of discharge from the hospital.

Evidence for Effectiveness of the Practice

One of the three trials found a statistically significant decrease in the incidence of VAP with CASS when compared to standard treatment, while a second study showed a strong trend. All three trials reported a statistically significant delay in the time to development of VAP, ranging from 48 hours to 8 days. Two trials found a decreased incidence of VAP caused by *Staphylococcus aureus* and *Hemophilus influenzae*, but no change was observed in the incidence of VAP caused by *Pseudomonas aeruginosa* or *Enterobacteriaceae*. No difference in mortality was observed in any of the trials.

Potential for Harm

There is minimal potential for harm to patients from the application of CASS and no adverse patient events were reported in over 150 patients.

Costs and Implementation

The cost and cost-effectiveness of CASS have not been examined. The direct costs appear minimal. Hi-Lo Evac tubes cost approximately 25% more than standard endotracheal tubes, putting the estimated cost of each unit at less than $1. The cost-savings per episode of VAP prevented could therefore be substantial. Implementation would largely be a matter of making the specialized endotracheal tubes available and providing staff training. The mechanical suctioning apparatus would require frequent monitoring by nursing or respiratory therapy to insure adequate function.

Comment

Continuous aspiration of subglottic secretions is a promising strategy for the prevention of VAP. Two randomized controlled trials have suggested a decrease in the rate of VAP in patients requiring prolonged (>3 days) mechanical ventilation (only one trial was statistically significant). The third trial showed no difference, but the patient population in this trial included many short-term intubations (mean duration of 36 hours) and was restricted to patients undergoing cardiac surgery. Larger randomized controlled trials are needed to address the impact of CASS more definitively. Another interesting observation is the delay in the development of VAP and the decreased incidence of *Staphylococcus aureus* and *Hemophilus influenzae*. This suggests that CASS may provide most of its benefit by preventing early VAP caused by community-acquired organisms, and its use could therefore be targeted to those patients requiring mechanical ventilation for intermediate periods of time (i.e., those at greatest risk for early VAP).

PREVENTION OF SURGICAL SITE INFECTIONS

Surgical site infections (SSI) include superficial incisional infections, infections of the deep incision space and organ space infections. A large body of evidence supports the premise that SSIs can be prevented through administration of appropriate prophylactic antibiotics. Two national organisations, the federal Centers for Disease Control and Prevention (CDC) and the American Society for Health System Pharmacists (ASHP), have recently synthesized this vast literature to produce comprehensive guidelines regarding the administration of prophylactic antibiotics across a broad range of procedures. Because of the breadth of this literature, we limited the focus of this review of strategies to prevent SSIs to adult surgery and procedures that typically occur in the operating room (as opposed to procedures such as endoscopy, interventional cardiology, or radiology procedures).

Practice Description

Antimicrobial prophylaxis refers to a brief course of an antimicrobial agent administered just before an operation begins in order to reduce intraoperative microbial contamination to a level that will not overwhelm host defenses and result in infection. To maximise the benefits of antimicrobial prophylactic, the agent used should be safe, inexpensive, and bactericidal with an *in vitro* spectrum that covers the most probable contaminants for the operation. Administration, usually by intravenous infusion, should be timed so that a bactericidal concentration is present in serum and tissues by the time the skin is incised. This practice is now standard of care and recommended by professional societies. Therapeutic levels in serum and tissues should be maintained until, at most, a few hours after the incision is closed in the operating room.

Prevalence and Severity of the Target Safety Problem

Surgical site infections are a common complication of care, occurring in 2-5% of patients after clean extra-abdominal surgeries (e.g., thoracic and orthopedic surgery) and in up to 20% of patients undergoing intra-abdominal procedures. Studies following patients into the post-discharge period have reported even higher rates of postoperative infection. These complications increase morbidity for patients and consume substantial additional resources.

Opportunities for Impact

Approximately 80-90% of surgical patients receive some kind of antibiotic prophylaxis, though recent studies have shown that choice of regimen, timing of administration or duration of prophylaxis is inappropriate in approximately 25-50% of cases.

Study Designs and Outcomes

As previously noted, the literature on prophylactic antibiotics is extensive. Therefore, the review was limited to evidence from Level 1A study designs. We identified 9 relevant studies examining the use of prophylactic antibiotics to prevent surgical site infections: 7 meta-analyses and 2 systematic reviews. These reviews were of high quality and limited their source material to randomized controlled trials. Although additional randomized trials have been published since these reviews were performed, updating the results of each review was beyond the scope of this project. All studies examined measured rates of site infection directly (Level 1), using previously published definitions to allow comparability. In addition, the rates of sepsis, length of stay, and physiologic measures were reported. One meta-analysis and one systematic review combined rates of several relevant infectious outcomes.

Evidence for Effectiveness of the Practice

All studies showed a marked reduction in the odds or relative risk of SSI when antibiotic prophylaxis was employed. None of the meta-analyses reviewed explicitly examined the timing of prophylaxis, although many studies pooled data from investigations of antibiotic regimens administered in the immediate preoperative period, (i.e., within minutes to an hour of initial incision). Two meta-analyses in our review suggested a trend towards lower rates of infection with use of broader-spectrum antibiotic prophylaxis, such as third generation cephalosporins. When compared with single dose prophylaxis, multiple dose prophylaxis generally did not result in significant additional benefit. In fact, Tanos et al found the odds of SSI were significantly less with single dose prophylaxis. Gillespie et al reported a greater relative risk of infection with single dose prophylaxis with a short-acting antibiotic when compared with multiple dose prophylaxis. However, the risk of infection with single dose prophylaxis using long-acting antibiotics did not differ significantly from that seen with multiple-dose regimens.

Potential for Harm

None of the meta-analyses analysed reported rates of adverse events (such as allergic reactions or nosocomial infections) associated with antibiotic prophylaxis of any type or duration. Both of the systematic reviews noted a trend towards more frequent adverse events with the use of antibiotic prophylaxis. Authors of both systematic reviews observed that these events were reported rarely and that variation in the definition of "adverse events" across studies made pooling results difficult.

Infection with *Clostridium difficile* affects a large number of hospitalized patients and has significant clinical and economic implications. As many as 16% of *C. difficile* colitis cases in surgical patients can be attributed to prophylaxis alone, with higher risk for this complication among patients receiving broad-spectrum antibiotics or prolonged courses of therapy. Shortening the duration of antibiotic administration may reduce potential risks of prophylaxis. Emergence of other types of resistant pathogens is an additional theoretical concern of inappropriate antibiotic prophylaxis; our literature search found no data describing effect of antibiotic prophylaxis on population-level incidence of these pathogens.

Costs and Implementation

A number of studies have evaluated strategies for improving compliance with recommended practices for perioperative antibiotic prophylaxis. These include chart audit with feedback, computerized decision support, dissemination of guidelines, total quality management (TQM) and continuous quality improvement (CQI) techniques, provider education programs, and comprehensive efforts by an infection control team. Another promising and easily implemented method is to delegate the administration of prophylactic antibiotics to the anesthesia team or the holding room nursing staff.

Costs for systems to increase appropriate use of antibiotics will likely be offset by savings due to prevented infections. However formal analyses of the cost-effectiveness of specific programs to improve prophylaxis have not been reported.

Comment

For many surgical procedures there is clear evidence supporting the use of antibiotic prophylaxis, administered in a timely manner, to prevent surgical site infections. The reviews suggest that broader spectrum antibiotics may be superior to limited-spectrum antibiotics for intra-abdominal or gynecologic surgeries. In addition, single-dose antibiotic prophylaxis appears to be at least as effective as multiple-dose regimens for a broad range of surgical procedures and may pose less risk to patients in terms of adverse events (e.g., *C. difficile* colitis) and less risk to the population in terms of microbial resistance. Future research will continue to address what prophylactic regimens are most effective for various surgical procedures. Investigation should also focus on methods to improve compliance. The optimal strategies for implementation will likely vary from institution to institution.

PNEUMOCOCCAL VACCINATION PRIOR TO HOSPITAL DISCHARGE

Streptococcus pneumoniae (pneumococcus) is a leading cause of serious community-acquired infections, especially pneumonia, the sixth leading cause of death in the United States. It causes over 50,000 cases of bacteremia and at least 500,000 cases of pneumonia annually in the United States. Although pneumococcus is an important pathogen in meningitis, bronchitis, and otitis media, these disease processes will not be discussed in this report.

The epidemiologic rationale for targeting pneumococcal vaccination among hospitalized patients derives from research showing that two-thirds of patients hospitalized with serious pneumococcal infections had been hospitalized at least once in the previous 3-5 years. One retrospective study showed that about 60% of persons 65 years of age and older hospitalized with pneumonia had been discharged from a hospital at least once in the prior 4 years. A prospective cohort study of patients aged 65 discharged from the hospital showed that the 5-year probability for readmission with pneumonia was over 7%. Hospitalisation, therefore, is a marker for patients at increased risk of developing subsequent pneumococcal infection. Despite the scope of the problem and the appeals for action from multiple specialty societies and national healthcare organisations, the vaccine is underutilized in the inpatient setting. This underutilisation has been attributed to uncertain effectiveness of the vaccine and ineffective methods of vaccine delivery during hospitalisation.

Hospital-based vaccination for patients at high risk of contracting pneumococcal infections is part of the action plan for adult immunisations developed by the federal Centers for Disease Control and Prevention (CDC) and the Health

Care Financing Administration (HCFA). It is also endorsed by the CDC's Advisory Committee on Immunisation Practices (ACIP) and the National Vaccine Advisory Committee. In addition, most national guidelines for the management of patients hospitalized with community-acquired pneumonia recommend vaccination against pneumococcus at time of discharge.

Practice Description

Currently, pneumococcal vaccines contain 23 capsular polysaccharide antigens of *S. pneumoniae* (23-valent vaccines). Over 88% of the serotypes that cause invasive disease in the United States, as well as 88% of serotypes accounting for penicillin-resistant isolates, are included in the 23-valent vaccine. Newer conjugate vaccines designed primarily to enhance the immune response in children are not covered in this review.

The practice of hospital-based pneumococcal vaccination is recommended for patients at increased risk for pneumococcal infection or increased risk of experiencing severe disease. Patients 65 years of age, or patients with certain chronic illnesses, including chronic cardiovascular disease, chronic pulmonary disease, diabetes, alcoholism, chronic liver disease, and functional or anatomic asplenia, are deemed high-risk. It is also recommended that all immunocompromised patients (due to HIV infection, leukemia, lymphoma, long term steroid use, or organ transplantation, among other causes) and any patient admitted with a diagnosis of community-acquired pneumonia be vaccinated. Vaccination could occur at any time during the hospitalisation, but is often recommended at discharge.

Prevalence and Severity of the Target Safety Problem

The goal of pneumococcal vaccination in hospitalized patients is to reduce the morbidity and mortality associated with pneumococcal infection, namely pneumococcal bacteremia and pneumococcal pneumonia. The CDC estimates the annual incidence of pneumococcal bacteremia at 15-30 cases per 100,000 population and 50-83 cases per 100,000 in persons aged 65. A recent study of the epidemiology of invasive *S. pneumoniae* (i.e., associated with bacteremia) in the United States found an overall incidence of 23.2 cases per 100,000, corresponding to 62,840 cases annually. The incidence among adults aged 65 and older was 59.7 per 100,000. The overall fatality rate was 10%, but patients aged 18-64 with an ACIP indication for vaccination had a fatality rate of 12.1%. Patients 65 years of age accounted for 51.4% of all deaths. These figures result in national estimates of over 6000 deaths in 1998 attributed to invasive pneumococcal disease.

The precise incidence of pneumococcal pneumonia is harder to estimate due to the poor sensitivity and specificity of diagnostic tests for this disease. At least 25-35% of all pneumonias are linked to *S. pneumoniae,* resulting in a minimum of 500,000 cases of pneumococcal pneumonia annually. Bacteremia complicates pneumococcal pneumonia in 10-25% of cases. The mortality rate for all patients hospitalized with community-acquired pneumonia is estimated at between 10-15%.

Opportunities for Impact

Despite recommendations to routinely vaccinate eligible hospitalized patients, pneumococcal vaccine is underutilized. The high potential impact of vaccination is borne out by recent epidemiologic evidence. Based on 1998 projections, 76% of invasive pneumococcal disease and 87% of deaths occur in patients who are eligible for pneumococcal vaccine. In addition, 88% of penicillin-resistant isolates during the same time period were of serotypes included in the 23-valent vaccine.

The vaccine is currently recommended for over 30 million persons aged 65 and over 23 million persons <65 who are at high risk. In 1997 only 45% of persons 65 and over reported ever receiving the vaccine. A 12-state study of Medicare patients hospitalized with pneumonia showed that the opportunity to provide the vaccine was missed in over 80% of patients, and only 0.4% of hospitalized elderly patients were vaccinated prior to discharge. More recent data from 1999 found a hospital vaccination rate in elderly patients screened, and not already vaccinated, of less than 9%. In this same study, vaccination rates were higher for patients with a discharge diagnosis of pneumonia (23.6%), but still far below the Public Health Service goal of 60%. Few data are available on rates of vaccination in patients <65 years of age who are otherwise at risk for pneumococcal infection.

In this chapter we considered two independent, but linked sets of studies: those evaluating the effectiveness of pneumococcal vaccination and those assessing strategies to increase vaccination rates in hospitalized patients. These two areas are reviewed separately below.

Vaccine Effectiveness

Study Designs and Outcomes

Three meta-analyses (published in 1994, 1999, and 2000) have analysed the effectiveness of pneumococcal vaccination in adults. The first study by Fine et al included 9 randomized controlled trials (RCTs) of vaccines (valences ranging from 6 to 17) in adults with and without risk factors for pneumococcal infection. Results were pooled and analysed for effects in various subgroups with careful attention to study heterogeneity (rate differences (RD) were reported when significant heterogeneity existed).

The second study included 13 randomized and quasi-randomized studies of vaccines with valences 2. Consequently, this study included 2 quasi-randomized studies with vaccine valences <6 that were excluded by Fine, but included a study by Austrian et al that was only partially included in the Fine meta-analysis. Results of this second meta-analysis were reported as pooled odds ratios; when significant heterogeneity existed, ranges were presented instead of pooled results.

The most recent meta-analysis identified 12 reports of 13 randomized controlled trials. The authors excluded 3 prior trial reports based on a predetermined decision to exclude quasi-randomized trials. Of these 3 quasi-randomized studies, the 2 older studies (26,000 patients) reported efficacy for the vaccine, while the more recent study (27,000 Finnish patients over aged 65) found no efficacy for pneumococcal vaccination. The 13 trials included 3 reports published after 1996 that were not included in either of the prior meta-analyses.

Despite the volume of RCTs that have been published, controversy still exists as to vaccine effectiveness in certain patient populations (high-risk, elderly), as wells as to the vaccine's effectiveness in reducing certain outcomes (pneumonia generally, and pneumococcal pneumonia). Consequently, we reviewed the 1997 summary report and recommendations of the Advisory Committee on Immunisation Practices, which synthesizes multiple case-control and cohort studies of vaccine effectiveness in high-risk patients. As an additional means to evaluate effectiveness, researchers from the CDC reported results of an indirect cohort analysis using a national database of pneumococcal bacteremia that compared distribution of pneumococcal serotypes causing infection in vaccinated and unvaccinated patients.

The 3 meta-analyses reported Level 1 outcomes, including

systemic pneumococcal infection and pneumococcal pneumonia. Two of these studies report infection rates with vaccine-type and non-vaccine-type organisms, and 2 of the 3 meta-analyses additionally report on all-cause pneumonia, bronchitis and mortality. All studies analyse data separately for elderly patients and high-risk patients, but the study by Hutchison et al differs from the other two with respect to this part of the analysis. In this study, vaccine efficacy in elderly and high-risk patients is assessed with logistic regression analysis after pooled odds ratios were determined, in contrast to the 2 other groups who report pooled odds ratios and relative risk separately for elderly, high-risk patients. The definition of pneumococcal pneumonia varied in many studies included in the pooled results, and in subsequent studies looking at the 23-valent vaccine. The indirect cohort analysis by Butler et al reported presumptive measures of effectiveness based on differing rates of isolation for certain serotypes of pneumococcus in vaccinated and unvaccinated patients (Level 2 outcome).

Evidence for Effectiveness of the Practice

The meta-analyses by Fine et al and Hutchison et al showed a protective effect of vaccination for systemic pneumococcal disease (66% effective overall, 83% effective against vaccine-types in the former; 73% effective overall, 83% effective against vaccine-types in the latter). Fine et al found the vaccine 53% effective for presumptive pneumococcal pneumonia, but analysis for heterogeneity showed that the rate difference was not statistically significant. The summary odds ratios for all other outcomes did not achieve statistical significance, either overall or in high-risk patients (i.e., patients age 55 years, patients with one or more chronic medical problems, and immunocompromised patients). Results for pneumococcal infection-related outcomes did achieve significance in low-risk patients.

Hutchison et al found effectiveness against pneumococcal pneumonia ranging from 31% to 76% (results were significant in 3 trials), but study heterogeneity prevented a pooled estimate. Regression analysis suggested similar benefits for systemic pneumococcal infection in elderly patients, but were inconclusive for systemic infection in chronically ill patients. For elderly patients, the authors estimated a number needed to treat (NNT) of 2520 to prevent a single case of pneumococcal bacteremia per year.

The most recent meta-analysis reported that in 3 comparisons involving approximately 21,100 immunocompetent subjects, pneumococcal vaccination was associated with significant reductions in the incidence of all-cause pneumonia (relative risk 0.56, 95% CI: 0.47-0.66), pneumococcal pneumonia (relative risk 0.16, 95% CI: 0.11-0.23), pneumonia deaths (relative risk 0.70, 95% CI: 0.50-0.96) and bacteremia (relative risk 0.18, 95% CI: 0.09-0.34). However, in 10 comparisons involving over 24,000 subjects who were elderly or likely to have impaired immune systems, the authors found no benefit to pneumococcal vaccination in terms of any clinical outcome of interest. While the relative risk for pneumococcal bacteremia in elderly or high-risk patients showed a trend towards benefit, the results were not statistically significant (relative risk 0.53, 95% CI: 0.14-1.94).

One additional publication has appeared since the search period covered by this most recent meta-analysis. This publication represents a 6-month preliminary report from a prospective comparison between 2 large cohorts (>100,000 subjects each) of Swedish patients age 65 years. Patients in one group received pneumococcal vaccine, influenza vaccine, or both. The other cohort consisted of all patients from the same region and age group who chose not to receive either of the vaccines. Among all vaccinated patients (results are pooled for pneumococcal and influenza vaccines), hospital admission for pneumonia (including all-cause pneumonia, pneumococcal pneumonia and invasive pneumococcal pneumonia) was significantly reduced, and overall mortality was reduced by 57% (95% CI: 55-60%). This study design has significant potential for bias, in that people who elect to participate in clinical studies tend to have better outcomes independent of the treatments they receive. Nonetheless, it seems unlikely that the results observed in this study, including a 57% reduction in all-cause mortality over a 6-month period, could be attributable solely to a selection effect tied to patients' decision to participate in the study.

4

Hospital Occupational Health and Safety

CONTROLLING OCCUPATIONAL EXPOSURE TO HAZARDOUS DRUGS

In response to numerous inquiries, OSHA published guidelines for the management of Cytotoxic (antineoplastic) drugs in the work place in 1986. At that time, surveys indicated little standardisation in the use of engineering controls and personal protective equipment (P.E.). Although practices improved in subsequent years, problems still exist. In addition, the occupational management of these chemicals has been further clarified. These trends, in conjunction with many information requests, have prompted OSHA to revise its recommendations for hazardous drug handling. Furthermore, some of these agents are covered under the Hazard Communication Standard (HCS) [29 CFR 1910.1200].

In order to provide recommendations consistent with current scientific knowledge, this informational guidance document has been expanded to cover hazardous drugs (HD), in addition to the cytotoxic drugs (CD) that were covered in the 1986 guidelines. The recommendations apply to all settings where employees are occupationally exposed to HD's, such as hospitals, physicians' offices and home health care agencies. It is recognized that sections dealing with work areas and prevention of employee exposure refer to workplaces where pharmaceuticals are used in concentrations appropriate for patient therapy. In those settings where employees work with drugs in a more potentially hazardous form, (e.g., a more concentrated form, encountered in certain components of pharmaceutical manufacturing), measures that afford employees a greater degree of protection from exposure are commonly employed and should be used.

This review will:

- Provide criteria for classifying drugs as hazardous.
- Summarize the evidence supporting the management of HD's as an occupational hazard.
- Discuss the equipment and worker education recommended as well as the legal requirements of standards for the protection of workers exposed and potentially exposed to HD's.
- Update the important aspects of medical surveillance.
- List some common HD's currently in use.

Anesthetic agents have not been considered in this review. However, exposure to some of these agents is a recognized health hazard, and a separate document on this topic is in the planning stage.

Categorisation Drugs as Hazardous

The purpose of this Paragraph is to describe the biological effects of those pharmaceuticals that are considered hazardous. A number of pharmaceuticals in the health care setting may pose occupational risk to employees through acute and chronic workplace exposure. Past attention had mainly focused on drugs used to treat cancer. However, it is clear that many other agents also have toxicity profiles of concern. This recognition prompted the American Society of Hospital Pharmacists (ASHP) to define a class of agents as "hazardous drugs". That report specified concerns about antineoplastic and non-antineoplastic hazardous drugs in use in most institutions throughout the country. OSHA shares this concern.

Characteristics

The ASHP Technical Assistance Bulletin (TAB) described four drug characteristics, each of which could be considered hazardous:

— genotoxicity;

— carcinogenicity;

— teratogenicity or fertility impairment; and

— serious organ or other toxic manifestation at low doses in experimental animals or treated patients.

Hazard Based on Pharmacology/Toxicology

Professional judgment by personnel trained in pharmacology/toxicology is essential in designating drugs as hazardous, and reference 65 provides information regarding the development of such a list at one institution. Some drugs, which have a long history of safe use in humans despite in vitro or animal evidence of toxicity, may be excluded by the institution's experts by considerations such as those used to formulate GRAS (Generally Regarded As Safe) lists by the FDA under the Food, Drug, and Cosmetics Act. In contrast, investigational drugs are new chemicals for which there is often little information on potential toxicity. Structure or activity relationships with similar chemicals and in vitro data can be considered in determining potential toxic effects. Investigational drugs should be prudently handled as HD's unless adequate information becomes available to exclude them.

Some major considerations by professionals trained in pharmacology/toxicology in designating a drug as hazardous are:

— Is the drug designated as Therapeutic Category 10:00 (Antineoplastic Agent) in the American Hospital Formulary Service Drug Information?

— Does the manufacturer suggest the use of special isolation techniques in its handling, administration, or disposal?

— Is the drug known to be a human mutagen, carcinogen, teratogen or reproductive toxicant?

— Is the drug known to be carcinogenic or teratogenic in animals (drugs known to be mutagenic in multiple bacterial systems or animals should also be considered hazardous)?

— Is the drug known to be acutely toxic to an organ system?

Hazardous Drugs ad Occupational Risks

Preparation, administration, and disposal of HD's may expose pharmacists, nurses, physicians, and other health care workers to potentially significant workplace levels of these chemicals. The literature establishing these agents as occupational hazards deals primarily with CD's; however, documentation of adverse exposure effects from other HD's is rapidly accumulating. The degree of absorption that takes place during work and the significance of secondary early biological effects on each individual encounter are difficult to assess and may vary depending on the HD. As a result, it is difficult to set safe levels of exposure on the basis of current scientific information. However, there are several lines of evidence supporting the toxic potential of these drugs if handled improperly. Therefore, it is essential to minimize exposure to all HD's. Summary tables of much of the data presented below can be found in Sorsa and Rogers.

Mechanism of Action

Most HD's either bind directly to genetic material in the cell nucleus or affect cellular protein synthesis. Cytotoxic drugs may not distinguish between normal and cancerous cells. The growth and reproduction of the normal cells are often affected during treatment of cancerous cells.

Animal Data

Numerous studies document the carcinogenic, mutagenic, and teratogenic effects of HD exposure in animals. They are well summarized in the pertinent IARC publications. Alkylating agents present the strongest evidence of carcinogenicity (e.g., cyclophosphamide, mechlorethamine hydrochloride [nitrogen mustard]). However, other classes, such as some antibiotics, have been implicated as well. Extensive evidence for mutagenic and reproductive effects can be found in all antineoplastic classes. The antiviral agent ribavirin has additionally been shown to be teratogenic in all rodent species tested. The ASHP recommends that all pharmaceutical agents that are animal carcinogens be handled as human carcinogens.

Human Data at Therapeutic Levels

Many HD's are known human carcinogens, for which there is no safe level of exposure. The development of secondary malignancies is a well-documented side effect of chemotherapy treatment. Leukemia has been most frequently observed. However, other secondary malignancies, such as bladder cancer and lymphoma, have been documented in patients treated for other, usually solid, primary malignancies.

Chromosomal aberrations can result from chemotherapy treatment as well. One study, on chlorambucil, reveals chromosomal damage in recipients to be cumulative and related to both dose and duration of therapy. Numerous case reports have linked chemotherapeutic treatment to adverse reproductive outcomes. Testicular and ovarian dysfunction, including permanent sterility, have occurred in male and female patients who have received CD's either singly or in combination. In addition, some antineoplastic agents are known or suspected to be transmitted to infants through breast milk.

The literature also documents the effects of these drugs on other organ systems. Extravasation of some agents can cause severe soft-tissue injury, consisting of necrosis and sloughing of exposed areas. Other HD's, such as pentamidine and zidovudine (formerly AZT), are known to have significant side effects (i.e., hematologic abnormalities), in treated patients. Serum transaminase elevation has also been reported in treated patients.

Occuapational Exposure: Airborne Levels

Monitoring efforts for cytotoxic drugs have detected measurable air levels when exhaust biological safety cabinets (BSC) were not used for preparation or when monitoring was performed inside the BSC. Concentrations of fluorouracil ranging from 0.12 to 82.26 ng/m have been found during monitoring of drug preparation without a BSC, implying an opportunity for respiratory exposure. Elevated concentrations of cyclophosphamide were found by these authors as well. Cyclophosphamide has also been detected on the HEPA filters of flow hoods used in HD preparation, demonstrating aerosolisation of the drug and an exposure opportunity mitigated by effective engineering controls.

A recent study has reported wipe samples of cyclophosphamide, one of the class I IARC carcinogens, on surfaces of work stations in an oncology pharmacy and outpatient treatment areas (sinks and countertops). Concentrations ranged from 0.005 to 0.035 mcg/cm, documenting opportunity for dermal exposure. Administration of drugs via aerosolisation can lead to measurable air concentrations in the breathing zone of workers providing treatment. Concentrations of up to 18 mcg/m have been found by personal air sampling of workers administering pentamidine. Similar monitoring for ribavirin has found concentrations as high as 316 mcg/m.

Occupational Exposure: Biological Evidence of a Absorption

1. Urinary Mutagenicity.

a. Falck et al. were the first to note evidence of mutagenicity in the urine of nurses who handled cytotoxic drugs. The extent of this effect increased over the course of the work week. With improved handling practices, a decrease in mutagenic activity was seen. Researchers have also studied pharmacy personnel who reconstitute antineoplastic drugs. These employees showed increasingly mutagenic urine over the period of exposure; when they stopped handling the drugs, activity fell within 2 days to the level of unexposed controls. They also found mutagenicity in workers using horizontal laminar flow BSC's that decreased to control levels with the use of vertical flow containment BSC's.

b. Other studies have failed to find a relationship between exposure and urine mutagenicity. Sorsa summarizes this information and discusses the factors, such as differences in urine collection timing and variations in the use of PPE, which could lead to disparate results. Differences may also be related to smoking status; smokers exposed to CD's exhibit greater urine mutagenicity than exposed nonsmokers or control smokers — suggesting contamination of the work area by CD's and some contribution of smoking to their mutagenic profile.

2. Urinary Thioethers are glutathione conjugated metabolites of alkylating agents, which have been evaluated as an indirect means of measuring exposure. Workers who handle cytotoxic drugs have been reported to have increased levels compared to controls and also have increasing thioether levels over a 5-day work week. Other studies of nurses who handle CD's and of treated patients have yielded variable results, which could be due to confounding by smoking, PPE, and glutathione-S-transferase activity.

3. Urinary Metabolites. Venitt assayed the urine of pharmacy and nursing personnel handling cisplatin and found platinum concentrations at or below the limit of detection for both workers and controls. Hirst found cyclophosphamide in the urine of two nurses who handled the drug, documenting worker absorption. (Hirst also documented skin absorption in human volunteers by using gas chromatography after topical application of the drug.) Urinary pentamidine recovery has also been reported in exposed health care workers.

Occupational Exposure Human Effects

Cytogenetic Effects

a. A number of studies have examined the relationship of exposure to CD's in the workplace to chromosomal aberrations. These studies have looked at a variety of markers for damage, including sister chromatid exchanges (SCE), structural aberrations (e.g., gaps, breaks, translocations), and micronuclei in peripheral blood lymphocytes. The results have been somewhat conflicting. Several authors found increases in one or more markers. Increased mutation frequency has been reported as well.

b. Other studies have failed to find a significant difference between workers and controls. Some researchers have found higher individual elevations or a relationship between the number of drugs handled and SCE's. These disparate results are not unexpected. The difficulties in quantitating exposure have resulted in different exposure magnitudes between studies; workers in several negative studies appear to have a lower overall exposure. In addition, differences in the use of PPE and work technique will alter absorption of CD's and resultant biologic effects.

c. Finally, techniques for SCE measurement may not be optimal. A recent study that looked at correlation of phosphoramide-induced SCE levels with duration of anticancer drug handling found a statistically significant correlation coefficient of zero. Taken together, the evidence indicates an excess of markers of mutagenic exposure in unprotected workers.

Reproductive Effects

a. Reproductive effects associated with occupational exposure to CD's have been well documented. Heinminki et al. found no difference in exposure between nurses who had spontaneous abortions and those who had normal pregnancies. However, the study group consisted of nurses who were employed in surgical or medical floors of a general hospital. When the relationship between CD exposure and congenital malformations was explored, the study group was expanded to include oncology nurses, among others, and an odds ratio of 4.7 was found for exposures of more than once per week. This observed odds ratio is statistically significant.

b. Selevan et al. found a relationship between CD exposure and spontaneous abortion in a case-control study of Finnish nurses. This well-designed study reviewed the reproductive histories of 568 women (167 cases) and found a statistically significant odds ratio of 2.3. Similar results were obtained in another large case-control study of French nurses, and a study of Baltimore-area nurses found a significantly higher proportion of adverse pregnancy outcomes when exposure to antineoplastic agents occurred during the pregnancy. The nurses involved in these studies usually prepared and administered the drugs. Therefore, workplace exposure of these groups of professionals to such products has been associated with adverse reproductive outcomes in several investigations.

Other Effects

a. Hepatocellular damage has been reported in nurses working in an oncology ward; the injury appeared to be related to intensity and duration of work exposure to CD's. Symptoms such as lightheadedness, dizziness, nausea, headache, and allergic reactions have also been described in employees after the preparation and administration of antineoplastic drugs in unventilated areas. In occupational settings, these agents are known to be toxic to the skin and mucous membranes, including the cornea.

b. Pentamidine has been associated with respiratory damage in one worker who administered the aerosol. The injury consisted of a decrease in diffusing capacity that improved after exposure ceased. The onset of bronchospasm in a pentamidine-exposed worker has also been reported. Employees involved in the aerosol administration of ribavirin have noted symptoms of respiratory tract irritation. A number of medications including psyllium and various antibiotics are known respiratory and dermal sensitizers. Exposure in susceptible individuals can lead to asthma or allergic contact dermatitis.

Work Areas

Risks to personnel working with HD's are a function of the drugs' inherent toxicity and the extent of exposure. The main routes of exposure are: inhalation of dusts or aerosols, dermal absorption, and ingestion. Contact with contaminated food or cigarettes represents the primary means of ingestion. Opportunity for exposure to HD's may occur at many points in the handling of these drugs.

Pharmacy or Other Preparation Areas

In large oncology centers, HD's are usually prepared in the pharmacy. However, in small hospitals, outpatient treatment areas, and physicians' offices they have been prepared by physicians or nurses without appropriate engineering controls and protective apparel. Many HD's must be reconstituted, transferred from one container to another, or manipulated before administration to patients. Even if care is taken, opportunity for absorption through inhalation or direct skin contact can occur.

Examples of manipulations that can cause splattering, spraying, and aerosolisation include:

— withdrawal of needles from drug vials;

— drug transfer using syringes and needles or filter straws;

— breaking open of ampules; and
— expulsion of air from a drug-filled syringe.

Evaluation of these preparation techniques, using fluorescent dye solutions, has shown contamination of gloves and the sleeves and chest of gowns.

Horizontal airflow work benches provide an aseptic environment for the preparation of injectable drugs. However, these units provide a flow of filtered air originating at the back of the work space and exiting toward the employee using the unit. Thus, they increase the likelihood of drug exposure to both the preparer and other personnel in the room. As a result, the use of horizontal BSC's is contra-indicated in the preparation of HD's. Smoking, drinking, applying cosmetics, and eating where these drugs are prepared, stored, or used also increase the chance of exposure.

Administration of Drugs to Patients

Administration of drugs to patients is generally performed by nurses or physicians. Drug injection into the IV line, clearing of air from the syringe or infusion line, and leakage at the tubing, syringe, or stopcock connection present opportunities for skin contact and aerosol generation. Clipping used needles and crushing used syringes can produce considerable aerosolisation as well.

Such techniques where needles and syringes are contaminated with blood or other potentially infectious material are prohibited by the Bloodborne Pathogens Standard. Prohibition of clipping or crushing of any needle or syringe is sound practice. Excreta from patients who have received certain antineoplastic drugs may contain high concentrations of the drug or its hazardous metabolites. For example, patients receiving cyclophosphamide excrete large amounts of the drug and its mutagenic metabolites.

Patients treated with cisplatin have been shown to excrete potentially hazardous amounts of the drug. Unprotected handling of urine or urine-soaked sheets by nursing or housekeeping personnel poses a source of exposure.

Disposal of Drugs and Contaminated Materials

Contaminated materials used in the preparation and administration of HD's, such as gloves, gowns, syringes and vials, present a hazard to support and housekeeping staff. The use of properly labeled, sealed and covered disposal containers, handled by trained and protected personnel, should be routine, and is required under the Bloodborne Pathogens Standard if such items are contaminated with blood or other potentially infectious materials. HD's and contaminated materials should be disposed of in accordance with federal, state, and local laws. Disposal of some of these drugs is regulated by the EPA. Drugs that are unused commercial chemical products and are considered by the EPA to be toxic wastes must be disposed of in accordance with 40 CFR part 261. Spills can also represent a hazard; the employer should ensure that all employees are familiar with appropriate spill procedures.

Survey of Current Work Practices

Surveys of U.S. cancer centers and oncology clinics reveal wide variation in work practices, equipment or training for personnel preparing CD's. This lack of standardisation results in a high prevalence of potential occupational exposure to CD's. One survey found that 40% of hospital pharmacists reported a skin exposure to CD's at least once a month, and only 28% had medical surveillance programmes in their workplaces.16 Nurses, particularly those in outpatient settings, were found to be even less well protected than pharmacists. Such findings emphasize current lack of protection for all personnel who risk potential exposure to HD's.

Prevention of Employee Exposure

Hazardous Drug Safety and Health Plan

Where hazardous drugs, as defined in this review, are used in the workplace, sound practice dictates that a written *Hazardous Drug Safety and Health Plan* be developed. Such a plan assists in:

— Protecting employees from health hazards associated with HD's.

— Keeping exposures as low as reasonably achievable.

When a *Hazardous Drug Safety and Health Plan* is developed, it should be readily available and accessible to all employees, including temporary employees, contractors, and trainees. The ASHP recommends that the Plan include each of the following elements and indicate specific measures that the employer is taking to ensure employee protection:

— Standard operating procedures relevant to safety and health considerations to be followed when health care workers are exposed to hazardous drugs.

— Criteria that the employer uses to determine and implement control measures to reduce employee exposure to hazardous drugs, including engineering controls, the use of personal protective equipment, and hygiene practices.

— A requirement that ventilation systems and other protective equipment function properly, and specific measures to ensure proper and adequate performance of such equipment.

— Provision for information and training.

— The circumstances under which the use of specific HD's (that is, FDA investigational drugs) require prior approval from the employer before implementation.

— Provision for medical examinations of potentially exposed personnel.

— Designation of personnel responsible for implementation of the *Hazardous Drug Safety and Health Plan* including the assignment of a Hazardous Drug Officer (who is an industrial hygienist, nurse, or pharmacist health and safety representative) and, if appropriate, establishment of a Hazardous Drug Committee or a joint Hazardous Drug Committee/ Chemical Committee.

The ASHP further recommends that specific consideration of the following provisions be included where appropriate:

— Establishment of a designated HD handling area.

— Use of containment devices such as biological safety cabinets.

— Procedures for safe removal of contaminated waste.

— Decontamination procedures.

The ASHP recommends that the *Hazardous Drug Safety and Health Plan* be reviewed and its effectiveness reevaluated at least annually and updated as necessary.

A comparison of OSHA 200 log entries to employee medical clinic appointment or visit rosters can be made to establish if there is evidence of disorders that could be related to hazardous drugs. Previous health and safety inspections by local health departments, fire departments, regulatory, or accrediting agencies may be helpful for the facility's planning purposes as well as any OSHA review of hazards and programmes in the facility. Joint Commission on Accreditation of Healthcare Organisations (JCAHO), or College of American Pathologists (CAP) review of facilities may contain information on hazardous drugs used in the facility.

Drug Preparatrion Precuations

Work Area

The ASHP recommends that HD preparation be performed in a restricted, preferably, centralized area. Signs restricting the access of unauthorized personnel are to be prominently displayed. Eating, drinking, smoking, chewing gum, applying cosmetics, and storing food in the preparation area should be prohibited. The ASHP recommends that procedures for spills and emergencies, such as skin or eye contact, be available to workers, preferably posted in the area.

Biological Safety Cabinets

Class II or III Biological Safety Cabinets (BSC) that meet the current National Sanitation Foundation Standard should minimize exposure to HD's during preparation. Although these cabinets are designed for biohazards, several studies have documented reduced urine mutagenicity in CD-exposed workers or reduced environmental levels after the institution of BSC's. If a BSC is unavailable, for example in private practice office, accepted practice is the sharing of a cabinet (e.g., several medical offices share a cabinet) or sending the patient to a center where HD's can be prepared in a BSC. Alternatively, preparation can be performed in a facility with a BSC and the drugs transported to the area of administration. Use of a dedicated BSC, where only HD's are prepared, is prudent practice.

Types Of BSC's

a. Four main types of Class II BSC's are available. They all have downward airflow and HEPA filters. They are differentiated by the amount of air recirculated within the cabinet, whether this air is vented to the room or the outside, and whether contaminated ducts are under positive or negative pressure. These four types are described below:

— Type A cabinets recirculate approximately 70% of cabinet air through HEPA filters back into the cabinet; the rest is discharged through a HEPA filter into the preparation room. Contaminated ducts are under positive pressure.

— Type B1 cabinets have higher velocity air inflow, recirculate 30% of the cabinet air, and exhaust the rest to the outside through HEPA filters. They have negative-pressure contaminated ducts and plenums.

— Type B2 systems are similar to Type B1 except that no air is recirculated.

— Type B3 cabinets are similar to Type A in that they recirculate approximately 70% of cabinet air. However, the other 30% is vented to the outside and the ducts are under negative pressure.

b. Class III cabinets are totally enclosed with gas tight construction. The entire cabinet is under negative pressure, and operations are performed through attached gloves. All air is HEPA filtered.

c. Class II, type B, or Class III BSC's are recommended since they vent to the outside. Those without air recirculation are the most protective. If the BSC has an outside exhaust, it should be vented away from air intake units.

d. The exhaust fan or blower on the vertical airflow hood should be on at all times, except when the hood is being mechanically repaired or moved. If the blower is turned off, the hood should be decontaminated before reuse. Each BSC should be equipped with a continuous monitoring device to allow confirmation of adequate air flow and cabinet performance. The cabinet should be in an area with minimal air turbulence; this will reduce leakage to the environment. Additional information on design and performance testing of BSC's can be found in papers by Avis and Levchuck, Bryan and Marback, and the National Sanitation Foundation. Practical information regarding space needs and use of BSC's is contained in the ASHP's 1990 technical assistance bulletin.

e. Ventilation and biosafety cabinets installed should be maintained and evaluated for proper performance in accordance with the manufacturer's instructions.

Decontamination

a. The cabinet should be cleaned according to the manufacturer's instructions. Some manufacturers have recommended weekly decontamination, as well as whenever spills occur, or when the cabinet requires moving, service or certification.

b. Decontamination should consist of surface cleaning with water and detergent followed by thorough rinsing. The use of detergent is recommended because there is no single accepted method of chemical deactivation for all agents involved. Quaternary ammonium cleaners should be avoided due to the possibility of vapor build-up in recirculated air. Ethyl alcohol or 70% isopropyl alcohol may be used with the cleaner if the contamination is soluble only in alcohol. Alcohol vapor build-up has also been a concern, so the use of alcohol should be avoided in BSC's where air is recirculated. Spray cleaners should also be avoided due to the risk of spraying the

HEPA filter. Ordinary decontamination procedures, which include fumigation with a germicidal agent, are inappropriate in a BSC used for HD's because such procedures do not remove or deactivate the drugs.

c. Removable work trays, if present, should be lifted in the BSC so the back and any sump below can be cleaned. During cleaning, the worker should wear PPE similar to that used for spills. *Ideally, the sash should remain down during cleaning, however, a NIOSH-approved respirator appropriate for the hazard must be worn by the worker if the sash will be lifted during the process.* The exhaust fan/blower should be left on. Cleaning should proceed from least to most contaminated areas. The drain spillage trough area should be cleaned at least twice since it can be heavily contaminated. All materials from the decontamination process should be handled as HD's and disposed of in accordance with federal, state, and local laws.

Service and Certification

a. The ASHP recommends that BSC's be serviced and certified by a qualified technician every six months or any time the cabinet is moved or repaired. Technicians servicing these cabinets or changing the HEPA filters should be aware of HD risks through hazard communication training from their employers and should use the same personal protective equipment as recommended for large spills.

b. Certification of the BSC includes performance testing as outlined in the procedures of the National Sanitation Foundation's Standard Number 49. Helpful information on such testing can be found in the ASHP 1990 technical assistance bulletins, the

BSC manufacturer's equipment manuals, and Bryan and Marback's paper. HEPA filters should be changed when they restrict airflow or if they are contaminated by an accidental spill. They should be bagged in plastic and disposed of as HD's. Any time the cabinet is turned off or transported it should be sealed with plastic.

Personal Protective Equipment

a. Gloves. Research indicates that the thickness of the gloves used in handling HD's is more important than the type of material, since all materials tested have been found to be permeable to some HD's. The best results are seen with latex gloves. Therefore, latex gloves should be used for the preparation of HD's unless the drug-product manufacturer specifically stipulates that some other glove provides better protection. Thicker, longer latex gloves that cover the gown cuff are recommended for use with HD's. Gloves with minimal or no powder are preferred since the powder may absorb contamination.

   The above referenced sources have noted great variability in permeability within and between glove lots. Therefore, double gloving is recommended if it does not interfere with an individual's technique. Because all gloves are permeable to some extent and their permeability increases with time, they should be changed regularly (hourly) or immediately if they are torn, punctured, or contaminated with a spill. Hands should always be washed before gloves are put on and after they are removed. Employees need thorough training in proper methods for contaminated glove removal.

b. Gowns. A protective disposable gown made of lint-free, low-permeability fabric with a closed front, long sleeves, and elastic or knit closed cuffs should be worn. The cuffs should be tucked under the gloves. If double gloves are worn, the outer glove should be over the gown cuff and the inner glove should be under the gown cuff. When the gown is removed, the inner glove should be removed last. Gowns and gloves in use in the HD preparation area should not be worn outside the HD preparation area.

As with gloves, there is no ideal material. Research has found nonporous Tyvek and Kaycel to be more permeable than Saranex-laminated Tyvek and polyethylene-coated Tyvek after four hours of exposure to the CD's tested. However, little airflow is allowed with the latter materials. As a result, manufacturers have produced gowns with Saranex or polyethylene reinforced sleeves and front in an effort to decrease permeability in the most exposure prone areas, but little data exists on decreasing exposure.

c. Respiratory Protection. A BSC is essential for the preparation of HD's. Where a BSC is not currently available, a NIOSH-approved respirator appropriate for the hazard must be worn to afford protection until the BSC is installed. *[NIOSH recommendation at the time of this publication is for a respirator with a high-efficiency filter, preferably a powered, air-purifying respirator.]* The use of respirators must comply with OSHA's Respiratory Protection Standard, which outlines the aspects of a respirator programme, including selection, fit testing, and worker training. Surgical masks are not appropriate since they do not prevent aerosol inhalation. Permanent respirator use, in lieu of BSC's, is imprudent practice and should not be a substitute for engineering controls.

d. Eye and Face Protection. Whenever splashes, sprays, or aerosols of HD's may be generated that can result in eye, nose, or mouth contamination, chemical-barrier face and eye protection must be provided and used in accordance with 29 CFR 1910.133. Eyeglasses with temporary side shields are inadequate protection.

   When a respirator is used to provide temporary protection as described above, and splashes, sprays, or aerosols are possible, employee protection should be:

   — a respirator with a full face piece; or

   — a plastic face shield or splash goggles complying with ANSI standards when using a respirator of less than full-face piece design.

e. PPE Disposal and Decontamination. All gowns, gloves, and disposable materials used in preparation should be disposed of according to the hospital's hazardous drug waste procedures and as described under this review's section on Waste Disposal. Goggles, face shields and respirators may be cleaned with mild detergent and water for reuse.

Work Equipment

NIH has recommended that work with HD's be carried out in a BSC on a disposable, plastic-backed paper liner. The liner should be changed after preparation is completed for the day or after a shift, whichever comes first. Liners should also be changed after a spill. Syringes and IV sets with Luer-lock fittings should be used for HD's. Syringe size should be large enough so that they are not full when the entire drug dose is present.

A covered disposable container should be used to contain excess solution. A covered sharps container should be in the BSC. The ASHP recommends that HD-labeled plastic bags be available for all contaminated materials (including gloves, gowns, and paper liners), so that contaminated material can be immediately placed in them and disposed of in accordance with ASHP recommendations.

Work Practices

Correct work practices are essential to worker protection. Aseptic technique is assumed as a standard practice in drug preparation. The general principles of aseptic technique, therefore, will not be detailed here. It should be noted, however, that BSC benches differ from horizontal flow units in several ways that require special precautions. Manipulations should not be performed close to the work surface of a BSC. Unsterilized items, including liners and hands, should be kept downstream from the working area.

Entry and exit of the cabinet should be perpendicular to the front. Rapid lateral hand movements should be avoided. Additional information can be found in the *National Sanitation Foundation Standard 49 for Class II (Laminar Flow) Biohazard Cabinetry* and Avis and Levchuck's paper. All operators should be trained in these containment area protocols. All PPE should be donned before work is started in the BSC. All items necessary for drug preparation should be placed within the BSC before work is begun. Extraneous items should be kept out of the work area.

a. Labeling. In addition to standard pharmacy labeling practices, all syringes and IV bags containing HD's should be labeled with a distinctive warning label, such as:

b. Needles. The ASHP recommends that all syringes and needles used in the course of preparation be placed in "sharps" containers for disposal without being crushed, clipped or capped.

c. Priming. Prudent practice dictates that drug administration sets be attached and primed within the BSC, prior to addition of the drug. This eliminates the need to prime the set in a less well-controlled environment and ensures that any fluid that escapes during priming contains no drug. If priming must occur at the site of administration, the intravenous line should be primed with non-drug containing fluid or a back-flow closed system should be used.

d. Handling Vials. Extremes of positive and negative pressure in medication vials should be avoided, e.g., attempting to withdraw 10 cc of fluid from a 10-cc vial or placing 10 cc of a fluid into an air-filled 10-cc vial. The use of large-bore needles, #18 or #20, avoids high-pressure syringing of solutions. However, some experienced personnel believe that large-bore needles are more likely to drip. Multiuse dispensing pins are recommended to avoid these problems. Venting devices such as filter needles or dispensing pins permit outside air to replace the withdrawn liquid. Proper worker education is essential before using these devices. Although venting devices are recommended, another technique is to add diluent slowly to the vial by alternately injecting small amounts and allowing displaced air to escape into the syringe. When all diluent has been added, a small amount of additional air may be withdrawn to create a slight negative pressure in the vial. This should not be expelled into room air because it may contain drug residue. It should either be injected into a vacuum vial or remain in the syringe to be discarded. If any negative pressure must be applied to withdraw a dosage from a stoppered vial and handling safety is compromised, an air-filled syringe should be used to equalize pressure in the stoppered vial. The volume of drug to be withdrawn can be replaced by injecting small amounts of air into the vial and withdrawing equal amounts of liquid until the required volume is withdrawn. The drug should be cleared from the needle and hub (neck) of the syringe before separating to reduce spraying on separation.

e. Handling Ampules. Prudent practice requires that ampules with dry material should be "gently tapped down" before opening to move any material in the top of the ampule to the bottom quantity. A sterile gauze pad should be wrapped around the ampule neck before breaking the top. This can protect against cuts and catch airborne powder or aerosol. If diluent is to be added, it should be injected slowly down the inside wall of the ampule. The ampule should be tilted gently to ensure that all the powder is wet before agitating it to dissolve the contents.

   After the solution is withdrawn from the ampule with a syringe, the needle should be cleared of solution by holding it vertically with the point upwards; the syringe should be tapped to remove air bubbles. Any bubbles should be expelled into a closed container.

f. Packaging HD's for Transport. The outside of bags or bottles containing the prepared drug should be wiped with moist gauze. Entry ports should be wiped with moist alcohol pads and capped. Transport should occur in sealed plastic bags and in containers designed to avoid breakage. Shipped HD's that are subject to EPA regulation as hazardous waste are also subject to Department of Transportation (DOT) regulations as specified in 49 CFR part 172.101.

g. Nonliquid HD's. The handling of nonliquid forms of HD's requires special precautions as well. Tablets which may produce dust or potential exposure to the handler should be counted in a BSC. Capsules, i.e., gel-caps or coated tablets, are unlikely to produce dust unless broken in handling. These are counted in a BSC on equipment designated for HD's only, because even manual counting devices may be covered with dust from the drugs handled. Automated counting machines should not be used unless an enclosed process isolates the hazard from the employee(s).

Compounding should also occur in a BSC. A gown and gloves should be worn. *(If a BSC is unavailable, an appropriate NIOSH-approved respirator must be worn.)*

Drug Administration

a. Personal Protective Equipment. The National Study Commission on Cytotoxic Exposure has recommended that personnel administering HD's wear gowns, latex gloves, and chemical splash goggles or equivalent safety glasses as described under the PPE section, preparation. *NIOSH-approved respirators should be worn when administering aerosolized drugs.*

b. Administration Kit. Protective and administration equipment may be packaged together and labeled as a HD administration kit. Such a kit could include:

— personal protective equipment;

— gauze (4" × 4") for cleanup;

— alcohol wipes;

— disposable plastic-backed absorbent liner;

— puncture-resistant container for needles and syringes;

— a thick sealable plastic bag (with warning label); and

— accessory warning labels.

c. Work Practices. Safe work practices when handling HD's should include the following:

— Hands should be washed before donning and after removing gloves. Gowns or gloves that become contaminated should be changed immediately. Employees should be trained in proper methods to remove contaminated gloves and gowns. After use, gloves and gowns should be disposed of in accordance with ASHP recommendations.

— Infusion sets and pumps, which should have Luer-lock fittings, should be observed for leakage during use. A plastic-backed absorbent pad should be placed under the tubing during administration to catch any leakage. Sterile gauze should be placed around any push sites; IV tubing connection sites should be taped.

— Priming IV sets or expelling air from syringes should be carried out in a BSC. If done at the administration site, ASHP recommends that the line be primed with non-drug containing solution or that a back-flow closed system be used. IV containers with venting tubes should not be used.

— Syringes, IV bottles and bags, and pumps should be wiped clean of any drug contamination with sterile gauze. Needles and syringes should not be crushed or clipped. They should be placed in a puncture-resistant container, then into the HD disposal bag with all other HD-contaminated materials.

— Administration sets should be disposed of intact. Disposal of the waste bag should follow HD disposal requirements. Unused drugs should be returned to the pharmacy.

— Protective goggles should be cleaned with detergent and properly rinsed. All protective equipment should be disposed of upon leaving the patient care area.

— Nursing stations where these drugs will be administered should have spill and emergency skin and eye decontamination kits available and relevant MSDS's for guidance. The HCS requires MSDS'S to be readily available in the workplace to all employees working with hazardous chemicals.

— PPE should be used during the administration of oral HD's if splashing is possible.

A large number of investigational HD's are under clinical study in health care facilities. Personnel not directly involved in the investigation should not administer these drugs unless they have received adequate instructions regarding safe handling procedures. Literature regarding potential toxic effects of investigational drugs should be evaluated prior to the drug's introduction into the workplace.

The increased use of HD's in the home environment necessitates special precautions. Employees involved in home care delivery should follow the above work practices and employers should make administration and spill kits available. Home health care workers should have emergency protocols with them as well as phone numbers and addresses in the event emergency care becomes necessary. Waste disposal for drugs delivered for home use and other home contaminated material should also be considered by the employer and should follow applicable regulations.

Aerosolized Drugs: The administration of aerosolized HD's requires special engineering controls to prevent exposure to health care workers and others in the vicinity. In the case of pentamidine, these controls include treatment booths with local exhaust ventilation designed specifically for its administration. A variety of ventilation methods have also been used for the administration of ribavirin. These include isolation rooms with separate HEPA filtered ventilation systems and administration via endotracheal tube. Engineering controls used to manage employee exposure to anesthetic gases is a traditional example of occupational chemical management. Both isolation and ventilation are used for these volatile HD's.

Caring for Patients Receiving HD's

In accordance with the Bloodborne Pathogens Standard, universal precautions must be observed to prevent contact with blood or other potentially infectious materials. Under circumstances in which differentiation between body fluid types is difficult or impossible, all body fluids should be considered potentially infectious materials and must be managed as dictated in the Bloodborne Pathogens Standard.

a. Personal Protective Equipment. Personnel dealing with excreta, primarily urine, from patients who have received HD's in the last 48 hours should be provided with and wear latex or other appropriate gloves and disposable gowns, to be discarded after each use or whenever contaminated, as detailed under Waste Disposal. Eye protection should be worn if splashing is possible. Such excreta contaminated with blood, or other potentially infectious materials as well, should be managed according to the Bloodborne Pathogen Standard. Hands should be washed after removal of gloves or after contact with the above substances.

b. Linen contaminated with HD's or excreta from patients who have received HD's in the past 48 hours is a potential source of exposure to employees. Linen soiled with blood or other potentially infectious materials as well as contaminated with excreta must also be managed according to the Bloodborne Pathogens Standard. Linen contaminated with HD's should be placed in specially marked laundry bags and then placed in a labeled impervious bag. The laundry bag and its contents should be prewashed, and then the linens added to other laundry for a second wash. Laundry personnel should wear latex gloves and gowns while handling prewashed material.

c. Reusable Items. Glassware or other contaminated reusable items should be washed twice with detergent by a trained employee wearing double latex gloves and a gown.

Waste Disposal

a. Equipment. Thick, leak-proof plastic bags, colored differently from other hospital trash bags, should be used for routine accumulation and collection of used containers, discarded gloves, gowns, and any other disposable material. Bags containing hazardous chemicals (as defined by Section C of HCS), shall be labeled in accordance with Section F of the Hazard Communication Standard where appropriate. Where the Hazard Communication Standard does not apply, labels should indicate that bags contain HD-related wastes. Needles, syringes, and breakable items not contaminated with blood or other potentially infectious materials should be placed in a "sharps" container before they are stored in the waste bag. Such items that *are* contaminated with blood or other potentially infectious material *must be* placed in a "sharps" container. Similarly, needles should not be clipped or capped nor syringes crushed if contaminated by blood or other potentially infectious material, except for a rare instance where a medical procedure requires recapping. The waste bag should be kept inside a covered waste container clearly labeled "HD WASTE ONLY." At least one such receptacle should be located in every area where the drugs are prepared or administered. Waste should not be moved from one area to another. The bag should be sealed when filled and the covered waste container taped.

b. Handling. Prudent practice dictates that every precaution be taken to prevent contamination of the exterior of the container. Personnel disposing of HD waste should wear gowns and protective gloves when handling waste containers with contaminated exteriors. Prudent practice further dictates that such a container with a contaminated exterior be placed in a second container in a manner that eliminates contamination of the second container. HD waste handlers should also receive hazard communication training as discussed below under Paragraph VIII: D of this chapter.

c. Disposal. Hazardous drug-related wastes should be handled separately from other hospital trash and disposed of in accordance with applicable EPA, state, and local regulations for hazardous waste. This disposal can occur at either an incinerator or a licensed sanitary landfill for toxic wastes, as appropriate. Commercial waste disposal is performed by a licensed company. While awaiting removal, the waste should be held in a secure area in covered, labeled drums with plastic liners.

Chemical inactivation traditionally has been a complicated process that requires specialized knowledge and training. The MSDS should be consulted regarding specific advice on cleanup. IARC and Lunn et al. have validated inactivation procedures for specific agents that are effective. However, these procedures vary from drug to drug and may be impractical for small amounts. Care must be taken because of unique problems presented by the cleanup of some agents, such as by-product formation. Serious consideration should be given to alternative disposal methods.

Spills

Emergency procedures to cover spills or inadvertent release of hazardous drugs should be included in the facility's overall health and safety programme. Incidental spills and breakages should be cleaned up immediately by a properly protected person trained in the appropriate procedures. The area should be identified with a warning sign to limit access to the area. Incident reports should be filed to document the spill and persons exposed.

a. Personnel Contamination. Contamination of protective equipment or clothing, or direct skin or eye contact should be treated by:

— Immediately removing the gloves or gown.

— Immediate cleansing of the affected skin with soap and water.

— Flooding an affected eye at an eyewash fountain or with water or isotonic eyewash designated for that purpose for at least 15 minutes, for eye exposure.

- Obtaining medical attention. (Protocols for emergency procedures should be maintained at the designated sites for such medical care. Medical attention should also be sought for inhalation of HD's in powder form.)
- Documenting the exposure in the employee's medical record.

b. Clean-up of Small Spills. The ASHP considers small spills to be those less than 5 ml. The 5-ml volume of material should be used to categorize spills as large or small. Spills of less than 5 ml or 5 gm outside a BSC should be cleaned up immediately by personnel wearing gowns, double latex gloves, and splash goggles. *An appropriate NIOSH-approved respirator should be used for either powder or liquid spills where airborne powder or aerosol is or has been generated.*

- Liquids should be wiped with absorbent gauze pads; solids should be wiped with wet absorbent gauze. The spill areas should then be cleaned three times using a detergent solution followed by clean water.
- Any broken glass fragments should be picked up using a small scoop (never the hands) and placed in a "sharps" container. The container should then go into a HD disposal bag, along with used absorbent pads and any other contaminated waste.
- Contaminated reusable items, for example glassware and scoops, should be treated as outlined above under Reusable Items.

c. Clean-up of Large Spills. When a large spill occurs, the area should be isolated and aerosol generation avoided. For spills larger than 5 ml, liquid spread is limited by gently covering with absorbent sheets or spill-control pads or pillows. If a powder is involved, damp cloths or towels should be used. Specific individuals should be trained to clean up large spills. Protective apparel, including respirators, should be used as with small spills when there is any suspicion of airborne powder or that an aerosol has been or will be generated. Most CD's are not volatile; however, this may not be true for all HD's. The volatility of the drug should be assessed in selecting the type of respiratory protection. As discussed under waste disposal, chemical inactivation should be avoided in this setting. All contaminated surfaces should be thoroughly cleaned three times with detergent and water. All contaminated absorbent sheets and other materials should be placed in the HD disposal bag.

d. Spills in BSC's. Extensive spills within a BSC necessitate decontamination of all interior BSC surfaces after completion of the spill cleanup. The ASHP recommends this action for spills larger than 150 ml or the contents of one vial. If the HEPA filter of a BSC is contaminated, the unit should be labeled and sealed in plastic until the filter can be changed and disposed of properly by trained personnel wearing appropriate protective equipment.

e. Spill Kits. Spill kits, clearly labeled, should be kept in or near preparation and administrative areas. The MSDS'S include sections on emergency procedures, including appropriate personal protective equipment. The ASHP recommends that kits include: chemical splash goggles, two pairs of gloves, utility gloves, a low-permeability gown, 2 sheets (12" × 12") of absorbent material, 250-ml and 1-liter spill control pillows, a “sharps” container, a small scoop to collect glass fragments, and two large HD waste-disposal bags.

Prior to cleanup, appropriate protective equipment should be donned. Absorbent sheets should be incinerable. Protective goggles and respirators should be cleaned with mild detergent and water after use.

Storage and Transport

a. Storage Areas. Access to areas where HD’s are stored should be limited to authorized personnel with signs restricting entry. A list of drugs covered by HD policies and information on spill and emergency contact procedures should be posted or easily available to employees. Optimally, facilities used for storing HD’s should not be used for other drugs, and such facilities should be designed to prevent containers from falling to the floor, e.g. bins with barrier fronts. Warning labels should be applied to all HD containers, as well as the shelves and bins where these containers are permanently stored.

b. Receiving Damaged HD Packages. Damaged shipping cartons should be opened in an isolated area or a BSC by a designated employee wearing double gloves, a gown, goggles, and appropriate respiratory protection. Individuals must be trained to process damaged packages as well. The ASHP recommends that broken containers and contaminated packaging mats be placed in a “sharps” container and then into HD disposal bags. The bags should then be closed and placed in receptacles, as described in the section on Waste Disposal. The appropriate protective equipment and waste disposal materials should be kept in the area where shipments are received, and employees should be trained in their use and the risks of exposure to HD's.

c. Transport. HD's should be securely capped or sealed, placed in sealed clear plastic bags, and transported in containers designed to avoid breakage. Personnel involved in transporting HD's should be trained in spill procedures, including sealing off the contaminated area and calling for appropriate assistance. All HD containers should be labeled as noted in *Drug Preparation Work Practices.* If transport methods that produce stress on contents (such as pneumatic tubes) are used, guidance from the OSHA clarification of 1910.1030 with respect to transport (M.4.b.(8)(c)) should be followed. This clarification provides for use of packaging material inside the tube to prevent breakage. These recommendations that pertain to the Bloodborne Pathogens Standard are prudent practice for HD's, e.g. padded inserts for carriers.

Medical Surveillance

Workers who are potentially exposed to chemical hazards should be monitored in a systematic programme of medical surveillance intended to prevent occupational injury and disease. The purpose of surveillance is to identify the earliest reversible biologic effects so that exposure can be reduced or eliminated before the employee sustains irreversible damage. The occurrence of exposure-related disease or other adverse health effects should prompt immediate re-evaluation of primary preventive measures (e.g., engineering controls, personal protective equipment). In this manner, medical surveillance acts as a check on the appropriateness of controls already in use.

For detection and control of work-related health effects,

job-specific medical evaluations should be performed, as follows:

— before job placement;
— periodically during employment;
— following acute exposures; and
— at the time of job termination or transfer (exit examination).

This information should be collected and analysed in a systematic fashion to allow early detection of disease patterns in individual workers and groups of workers.

Pre-Placement Medical Examinations

Sound medical practice dictates that employees who will be working with HD's in the workplace have an initial evaluation consisting of a history, physical exam, and laboratory studies. Information made available, by the employer, to the examining physician should be:

— A description of the employee's duties as they relate to the employee's exposure.
— The employee's exposure levels or anticipated exposure levels.
— A description of any personal protective equipment used or to be used.
— Information from previous medical examinations of the employee, which is not readily available to the examining physician.

The history details the individual's medical and reproductive experience with emphasis on potential risk factors, such as past hematopoietic, malignant, or hepatic disorders. It also includes a complete occupational history with information on extent of past exposures (including environmental sampling data, if possible) and use of protective equipment. Surrogates for worker exposure, in the absence of environmental sampling data, include:

— records of drugs and quantities handled;
— hours spent handling these drugs per week; and
— number of preparations/administrations per week.

The physical examination should be complete, but the skin, mucous membranes, cardiopulmonary and lymphatic systems, and liver should be emphasized. An evaluation for respirator use must be performed in accordance with 29 CFR 1910.134, if the employee will wear a respirator. The laboratory assessment may include a complete blood count with differential, liver function tests, blood urea nitrogen, creatinine, and a urine dipstick. Other aspects of the physical and laboratory evaluation should be guided by known toxicities of the HD of exposure. Due to poor reproducibility, interindividual variability, and lack of prognostic value regarding disease development, no biological monitoring tests (e.g., genotoxic markers) are currently recommended for routine use in employee surveillance. Biological marker testing should be performed only within the context of a research protocol.

Periodic Medical Examinations

Recognized occupational medicine experts in the HD area recommend these exams to update the employee's medical, reproductive, and exposure histories. They are recommended on a yearly basis or every two to three years. The interval between exams is a function of the opportunity for exposure, duration of exposure, and possibly the age of the worker at the discretion of the occupational medicine physician, guided by the worker's history. Careful documentation of an individual's routine exposure and any acute accidental exposures are made. The physical examination and laboratory studies follow the format outlined in the preplacement examination.

Post-exposure Examinations

Postexposure evaluation is tailored to the type of exposure (e.g., spills or needle sticks from syringes containing HD's). An assessment of the extent of exposure is made and included in the confidential database (discussed below) and in an incident report. The physical examination focuses on the involved area as well as other organ systems commonly affected (i.e. for CD's the skin and mucous membranes; for aerosolized HD's the pulmonary system). Treatment and laboratory studies follow as indicated and should be guided by emergency protocols.

Exit Examinations

The exit examination completes the information on the employee's medical, reproductive and exposure histories. Examination and laboratory evaluation should be guided by the individual's history of exposures and follow the outline of the periodic evaluation.

Exposure-Health Outcome Linkage

Exposure assessment of all employees who have worked with HD's is important, and the maintenance of records is required by 29 CFR 1910.1020. The use of previously outlined exposure surrogates is acceptable, although actual environmental or employee monitoring data is preferable. An MSDS can serve as an exposure record. Details of the use of personal protective equipment and engineering controls present should be included. A confidential database should be maintained with information regarding the individual's medical and reproductive history, with linkage to exposure information to facilitate epidemiologic review.

Reproductive Issues

The examining physician should consider the reproductive status of employees and inform them regarding relevant reproductive issues. The reproductive toxicity of hazardous drugs should be carefully explained to all workers who will be exposed to these chemicals, and is required for those chemicals covered by the HCS. Unfortunately, no information is available regarding the reproductive risks of HD handling with the current use of BSC's and PPE. However, as discussed earlier, both spontaneous abortion and congenital malformation excesses have been documented among workers handling some of these drugs without currently recommended engineering controls and precautions. The facility should have a policy regarding reproductive toxicity of HD's and worker exposure in male and female employees and should follow that policy.

Hazard Communication

This paragraph is for informational purposes only and is not a substitute for the requirements of the Hazard Communication Standard.

Discussion

The Hazard Communication Standard (HCS) is applicable to some drugs. It defines a hazardous chemical as any chemical that is a physical hazard or a health hazard. Physical hazard refers to characteristics such as combustibility or reactivity. A health hazard is defined as a chemical for which there is statistically significant evidence based on at least one study conducted in accordance with established scientific principles that acute or chronic health effects may occur in exposed employees. Appendixes A and B of the HCS outline the criteria used to determine whether an agent is hazardous.

According to HCS, agents with any of the following characteristics are considered hazardous:

— Carcinogens;
— Corrosives;
— Toxic or highly toxic (defined on the basis of median lethal doses);
— Irritants;
— Sensitizers; and
— Target organ effectors, including reproductive toxins, hepatotoxins, nephrotoxins, neurotoxins, agents that act on the hematopoietic system, and agents that damage the lungs, skin, eyes, or mucous membranes

Both human and animal data are to be used in this determination. HCS Appendix C lists sources of toxicity information.

As a result of the February 21, 1990, Supreme Court decision, all provisions of the HCS [29 CFR 1910. 1200] are now in effect for all industrial segments. This includes the coverage of drugs and pharmaceuticals in the non-manufacturing sector. On February 9, 1994, OSHA issued a revised Hazard Communication Final Rule with technical clarification regarding drugs and pharmaceutical agents. The HCS requires that drugs posing a health hazard (with the exception of those in solid, final form for direct administration to the patient, i.e., tablets or pills) be included on lists of hazardous chemicals to which employees are exposed. Their storage and use locations can be confirmed by reviewing purchasing office records of currently used and past used agents such as those in Appendix VI:2-1. Employee exposure records, including workplace monitoring, biological monitoring, and MSDS's as well as employee medical records related to drugs posing a health hazard must be maintained and access to them provided to employees in accordance with 29 CFR 1910.1020. Training required under the HCS should include all employees potentially exposed to these agents, not only health care professional staff, but also physical plant, maintenance, or support staff.

MSDS's are required to be prepared and transmitted with the initial shipment of all hazardous chemicals including covered drugs and pharmaceutical products. This excludes drugs defined by the Federal Food, Drug, and Cosmetic Act that are in solid, final form for direct administration to the patient (e.g. tablets, pills, or capsules) or that are packaged for sale to consumers in a retail establishment. Package inserts and the Physician's Desk Reference are not acceptable in lieu of requirements of MSDS's under tne Standard. Items mandated by the Standard will use the term shall instead of should.

Written Hazard Communication Programme

Employers shall develop, implement, and maintain at the workplace a written hazard communication programme for employees handling or otherwise exposed to chemicals, including drugs that represent a health hazard to employees. The written programme will describe how the criteria specified in the Standard concerning labels and other forms of warning, MSDS's, and employee information and training will be met. This also includes the following:

— A list of the covered hazardous drugs known to be present using an identity that is referenced on the appropriate MSDS.

— The methods the employer will use to inform employees of the hazards of nonroutine tasks in their work areas.

— The methods the employer will use to inform

employees of other employers of hazards at the work site.

The employer shall make the written hazard communication programme available, upon request, to employees, their designated representatives, and the Assistant Secretary of OSHA in accordance with requirements of the HCS.

MSDS's. In accordance with requirements in the Hazard Communication Standard, the employer must maintain MSDS's accessible to employees for all covered HD's used in the hospital. Specifics regarding MSDS content are contained in the Standard. Essential information includes: health hazards, primary exposure routes, carcinogenic evaluations, acute exposure treatment, chemical inactivators, solubility, stability, volatility, PPE required, and spill procedures for each covered HD. MSDS's shall also be made readily available upon request to employees, their designated representatives, or the Assistant Secretary of OSHA.

Training and Information Dissemination

Discussion

In compliance with the Hazard Communication Standard, all personnel involved in any aspect of the handling of covered HD's (physicians, nurses, pharmacists, housekeepers, employees involved in receiving, transport or storage) must receive information and training to appraise them of the hazards of HD's present in the work area. Such information should be provided at the time of an employee's initial assignment to a work area where HD's are present and prior to assignments involving new hazards. The employer should provide annual refresher information and training. The National Study Commission on Cytotoxic Exposure has recommended that knowledge and competence of personnel be evaluated after the first orientation or training session, and then yearly, or more often if a need is perceived. Evaluation may involve direct observation of an individual's performance on the job. In addition, non-HD solutions should be used for evaluation of preparation technique; quinine, which will fluoresce under ultraviolet light, provides an easy mechanism for evaluation of technique.

Employee Information

Employees must be informed of the requirements of the Hazard Communication Standard, 29 CFR 1910.1200, as follows:

- — Any operation/procedure in their work area where drugs that present a hazard are present.
- — The location and availability of the written hazard communication programme.
- — Any operations or procedure in their work area where other HD's are present.
- — The location and availability of any other plan regarding HD's.

Employee Training

Employee training must include at least the following elements:

- — Methods and observations that may be used to detect the presence or release of an HCS-covered hazardous drug in the work area (such as monitoring conducted by the employer, continuous monitoring devices, visual appearance or odor of covered HD's being released, etc.).
- — The physical and health hazards of the covered HD's in the work area.

— The measures employees can take to protect themselves from these hazards. This includes specific procedures that the employer has implemented to protect the employees from exposure to such drugs, such as identification of covered drugs and those to be handled as hazardous, appropriate work practices, emergency procedures (for spills or employee exposure).

— Personal protective equipment, and the details of the hazard communication programme developed by the employer, including an explanation of the labeling system and the MSDS, and how employees can obtain and use the appropriate hazard information.

It is essential that workers understand the carcinogenic potential and reproductive hazards of these drugs. Both females and males should understand the importance of avoiding exposure, especially early in pregnancy, to the drugs, so that they can make informed decisions about the hazards involved. In addition, the facility's policy regarding reproductive toxicity of HD's should be explained to workers. Updated information should be provided to employees on a regular basis and whenever their jobs involve new hazards. Medical staff and other personnel who are not hospital employees should be informed of hospital policies and of the expectation that they will comply with these policies.

Record-keeping

Any workplace exposure record created in connection with HD handling shall be kept, transferred, and made available for at least 30 years and medical records shall be kept for the duration of employment plus 30 years in accordance with the Access to Employee Exposure and Medical Records Standard (29 CFR 1910.1020). In addition, sound practice dictates that training records should include the following information:

— Dates of the training sessions;

— Contents or a summary of the training sessions;

— Names and qualifications of the persons conducting the training; and

— Names and job titles of all persons attending the training sessions.

Training records should be maintained for three years from the date on which the training occurred.

APPENDIX 1: SOME COMMON DRUGS THAT ARE CONSIDERED HAZARDOUS

Appendix 1 is not all-inclusive, should not be construed as complete, and represents an assessment of some, but not all, marketed drugs at a fixed point in time. Appendix VI:2-1 was developed through consultation with institutions that have assembled teams of pharmacists and other health care personnel to determine which drugs should be handled with caution. These teams reviewed product literature and drug information when considering each product.

Sources for this appendix are the "Physicians Desk Reference," Section 10:00 in the *American Hospital Formulary Service Drug Information*, IARC publications (particularly Volume 50), the Johns Hopkins Hospital, and the National Institutes of Health, Clinical Center Nursing Department. No attempt to include investigational drugs was made, but they should be prudently handled as hazardous drugs until adequate information becomes available to exclude them.

Any determination of the hazard status of a drug should be periodically reviewed and updated as new information becomes available. Importantly, new drugs should routinely undergo a hazard assessment.

Chemical / Generic Name	*Source**
ALTRETAMINE	C
AMINOGLUTETHIMIDE	A
AZATHIOPRINE	ACE
L-ASPARAGINASE	ABC
BLEOMYCIN	ABC
BUSULFAN	ABC
CARBOPLATIN	ABC
CARMUSTINE	ABC
CHLORAMBUCIL	ABCE
CHLORAMPHENICOL	E
CHLOROTIANISENE	B
CHLOROZOTOCIN	E
CYCLOSPORIN	E
CISPLATIN	ABCE
CYCLOPHOSPHAMIDE	ABCE
CYTARRABINE	ABC
DACARBAZINE	ABC
DACTINOMYCIN	ABC
DAUNORUBICIN	ABC
DIETHYLSTILBESTROL	BE
DOXORUBICIN	ABCE
ESTRADIOL	B
ESTRAMUSTINE	AB
ETHINYL ESTRADIOL	B
ETOPOSIDE	ABC
FLOXURIDINE	AC

FLUOROURACIL	ABC
FLUTAMIDE	BC
GANCICLOVIR	AD
HYDROXYUREA	ABC
IDARUBICIN	AC
IFOSFAMIDE	ABC
INTERFERON-A	BC
ISOTRETINOIN	D
LEUPROLIDE	BC
LEVAMISOLE	C
LOMUSTINE	ABCD
MECHLORETHAMINE	BC
MEDROXYPROGESTERONE	B
MEGESTROL	BC
MELPHALAN	ABCE
MERCAPTOPURINE	ABC
METHOTREXATE	ABC
MITOMYCIN	ABC
MITOTANE	ABC
MITOXANTRONE	ABC
NAFARELIN	C
PIPOBROMAN	C
PLICAMYCIN	BC
PROCARBAZINE	ABCE
RIBAVIRIN	D
STREPTOZOCIN	AC
TAMOXIFEN	BC
TESTOLACTONE	BC
THIOGUANINE	ABC

THIOTEPA	ABC
URACIL MUSTARD	ACE
VIDARABINE	D
VINBLASTINE	ABC
VINCRISTINE	ABC
ZIDOVUDINE	D

* Sources

A - The National Institutes of Health, Clinical Center Nursing Department

B - Antineoplastic drugs in the [italicize the following text name] Physicians' Desk Reference

C - American Hospital Formulary, Antineoplastics

D - Johns Hopkins Hospital

E - International Agency for Research on Cancer

APPENDIX 2: SOME AEROSOLIZED DRUGS

Ribavirin

Ribavirin is a synthetic nucleoside with antiviral activity against respiratory syncytial virus (RSV). It appears to restrict synthesis of viral proteins by interfering with mRNA production, but the exact mechanism of action remains unknown. It is reconstituted from a lyophilized powder for aerosol administration.

Ribavirin is usually administered in the aerosolized form via mask or oxygen tent for 12-18 hours per day for 3 to 7 days. A small particle aerosol generator (SPAG) creates respirable particles of 1.3 micrometer median diameter. Under current practice, excess drug is exhausted into the patient's room, causing additional exposures.

Studies have shown Ribavirin to be teratogenic in rodents and embryolethal in rabbits. Ribavirin induces cell transformation in an in-vitro mammalian system (Balb/C

3T3 cell line). In vivo carcinogenicity studies are incomplete.

Human studies on nurses who administer the drug by oxygen tent calculate that the absorbed dose of ribavirin per workshift is 13.5 mg/kg. This estimated dose exceeded 1/100 (the safety factor) of the short term daily dose levels toxic in animal models described above. No symptoms were reported by any health care worker in this study. However, minor pulmonary function abnormalities have been seen among healthy adult volunteers in clinical studies.

Pentamidine

Aerosolized pentamidine isethionate (4,4'-diamidinophenoxypentane) is FDA-approved for the treatment and prophylaxis of pneumonia caused by the protozoan *Pneumocystis carinii.* The exact mode of action is not fully understood; some studies indicate that pentamidine interferes with nuclear metabolism, inhibiting the synthesis of DNA, RNA, phospholipids, and proteins. It possesses two amidine groups and resembles other compounds called electrophiles which form DNA adducts. Pentamidine is administered as an aerosol after being reconstituted from a lyophilized powder.

No studies have been performed to evaluate the potential carcinogenic, mutagenic, or reproductive effects of pentamidine in animals or humans. Studies among health care workers have demonstrated pentamidine uptake by those personnel who administer the drug. Side effects include coughing, sneezing, mucous membrane irritation, headache, and bronchospasm. Pulmonary function tests have demonstrated transitory decreases in carbon monoxide diffusing capacity (DLCO). However, one respiratory therapist followed for 14 months has not returned to baseline after exposure

ULTRASOUND GUIDANCE OF CENTRAL VEIN CATHETERIZATION

The multiple indications for central venous catheters (CVCs) include parenteral nutrition, intravascular depletion, access for vasoactive medications, hemodynamic monitoring, cardiopulmonary arrest, difficult peripheral intravenous (IV) access and long-term IV access for medications, such as antibiotics. While these catheters can be life saving, they are also associated with significant risks. These risks increase in association with several characteristics, including patient anatomy (e.g., morbid obesity, cachexia, or local scarring from surgery or radiation treatment), patient setting (e.g., patients receiving mechanical ventilation or during emergencies such as cardiac arrest) and co-morbidities (e.g., bullous emphysema or coagulopathy).

CVCs are placed by clinicians whose training and experience may vary greatly. The procedure takes place in a variety of hospital settings including intensive care units, emergency departments, operating rooms, pre- and post-anesthesia care units, hemodialysis units, cardiac catheterisation units and other inpatient settings. Outpatient placement of CVCs has also become commonplace, occurring in hemodialysis centers and oncology centers providing outpatient chemotherapy.

Percutaneous insertions of CVCs are usually performed by "blind" techniques that rely on anatomic landmarks—i.e., palpable or visible structures with known relationships to the desired vein. For example, the infraclavicular approach to the subclavian vein requires correct localisation of the clavicle reference site, suprasternal notch and sternocleidomastoid-clavicular triangle landmarks, proper positioning of the patient and operator and correct venipuncture point depth, direction and insertion angle.

Analogously, the various approaches to the internal jugular vein require thorough knowledge of this vein's course in relation to the sternocleidomastoid muscle and carotid artery.

Newer technologies, such as portable ultrasound (US) devices, provide bedside imaging of the central veins during catheter placement. The advantages associated with US guided CVC placement include detection of anatomic variations and exact vessel location, avoidance of central veins with pre-existing thrombosis that may prevent successful CVC placement, and guidance of both guidewire and catheter placement after initial needle insertion. This review assesses the impact of real-time ultrasound guidance on improving the safety of CVC insertions.

Practice Description

Real-time ultrasound guidance of CVC insertion provides the operator with visualisation of the desired vein and the surrounding anatomic structures prior to and during insertion of the needle, guidewire and catheter. Previous studies of US location of vessels *followed* by subsequent catheter placement with landmark techniques found no advantages over standard landmark techniques. Real-time US guidance, on the other hand, appears to improve the success rate and decrease the complication rate associated with CVC placement. Two types of real-time ultrasound guidance are described. The Doppler US guidance method include audio-guided Doppler, fingertip pulsed Doppler and probe-in-the-needle technology. The non-Doppler US guidance methods (subsequently referred to as US guidance) includes US with needle guidance or without needle guidance.

Prevalence and Severity of the Target Safety Problem

The annual number of all CVCs insertions in the United States is not known, but is estimated at "several million" for subclavian-vein catheters. When aggregated with the various types of catheters placed into the central venous circulation and the increasing utilisation of CVCs among routine surgical patients, critically ill patients (in both emergency departments and intensive care units), and for the management of many patients undergoing hemodialysis or chemotherapy, the total number of CVC placements may be many times greater than estimates for subclavian CVCs alone.

Unsuccessful insertion of CVCs may occur in up to 20% of cases. The hazards associated with attempted CVC insertion (whether successful or not) include arterial puncture, hematoma, pneumothorax, hemothorax, chylothorax, brachial plexus injury, arrhythmias, air embolus, catheter malposition and catheter knotting. Other complications associated with CVCs, such as infection, thrombosis, arterial-venous fistula and vascular or cardiac erosion, are not usually associated with needle insertion but occur after catheter placement.

The frequency of complications associated with CVC placement is quite variable, largely due to differences among selected venous insertion sites, the degree of prior operator experience and the presence of previously described risk factors. In general, the rate of major CVC complications (e.g., pneumothorax or vessel laceration requiring repair) and minor complications (e.g., arterial puncture without significant hemorrhage, transient catheter malposition) is between 0.5 and 10%.

In addition to complications, several quality-of-care issues are associated with problems in CVC insertion. For example, a CVC insertion that requires multiple attempts may engender considerable patient anxiety and discomfort. More importantly, a prolonged insertion process may delay the infusion of life-saving fluids or medications during an emergency.

Opportunities for Impact

The majority of CVC insertions are placed using the landmark method. As set forth above, the number of catheters placed annually and the proportion currently inserted without US guidance is not known. Also unknown is the proportion of catheters placed in those patients who may benefit most from the US technique—those with multiple risk factors, those in high risk settings such as the intensive care unit, or those undergoing catheter placement by inexperienced operators. There are a variety of catheters that require access to the central veins. These include single and multi-lumen CVCs, tunneled and non-tunneled catheters, and larger, more rigid catheter introducers that permit passage of thinner, more flexible devices (e.g., pulmonary artery catheters, diagnostic cardiac catheters and temporary transvenous pacemakers). All centrally-placed catheters require an initial needle insertion into the vein, followed by a guidewire to permit passage of the catheter.

Study Designs

One meta-analysis and 10 original studies were analysed. Among the 10 original studies, 9 were randomized control studies and 1 study was a quasi-randomized control trial. The meta-analysis includes 6 references cited in this chapter. Four articles cited in this chapter were not cited in the 1996 meta-analysis, including 3 that were published after 1996 and one that included a quasi-randomized design. Two studies included in the meta-analysis were not included in this chapter because they were from non-English language journals.

All of the studies analysed for this chapter were prospective, non-blinded and randomized, with the exception of a quasi-randomized design involving alternate week allocation of patients to receive the intervention.

Randomisation was at the patient (rather than physician) level in all studies. The 10 original studies include 5 using an ultrasound guidance technique without Doppler and 5 using the Doppler US technique. Sites of catheterisation included the internal jugular (IJ) veins in 6 studies, the subclavian (SC) veins in 3 studies and the femoral veins in 1 study. The study populations are diverse and include intensive care unit patients, surgical patients both preoperatively and intraoperatively, cardiac patients in both the catheterisation and coronary care units, emergency department patients in cardiopulmonary arrest and oncology center outpatients.

Examples of studies excluded from analysis are studies lacking comparison control groups, studies of US use but without real-time guidance, and simulations of CVC placement rather than completed procedures.

Study Outcomes

Studies included for review reported a combination of clinical outcomes. These outcomes include Level 1 complications that resulted in increased patient morbidity (e.g., pneumothorax) and Level 2 complications that represent potential adverse events (e.g., unwanted arterial puncture without sequelae). Most studies also reported the number of venipuncture attempts to achieve successful CVC placement as well as the time required to complete successful CVC insertions. These are considered Level 2 outcomes because increased venipuncture attempts are associated with increased complication rates.

Evidence for Effectiveness of the Practice

The 1996 meta-analysis estimated that real-time US guidance for CVC insertion is associated with a significant reduction in placement failures as compared with the usual landmark techniques (relative risk 0.32, 95% CI: 0.18-0.55).

In addition, this review estimated that US guidance results in decreased complications during attempted CVC placements (relative risk 0.22, 95% CI: 0.10-0.45), corresponding to a relative risk reduction of 78%. The mean number of attempted venipunctures till successful CVC insertion was significantly reduced with real-time US guidance (relative risk 0.60, 95% CI: 0.45-0.79), corresponding to a relative risk reduction of 40%. Two of the 3 studies reviewed for this chapter and not included in the meta-analysis (because they were published subsequently) deserve mention because of contrary findings. Both 1998 studies included operators with significant prior experience placing CVCs by the usual landmark method. The overall failure rate for both landmark and US guidance techniques was very low in one study. The other study found statistically insignificant negative results associated with US guidance, owing to a high failure rate during the initial learning period for the newly-introduced US guidance technique, and a very low (1.3%) overall complication rate for CVC placement.

With the exception of femoral venous catheterisation during cardiopulmonary resuscitation, the studies reviewed for this chapter did not find reductions in insertion time when using real-time US guidance. With 2 exceptions, the cited studies reached statistical significance for at least one of the 3 outcome measures (morbidity, potential adverse events, and number of venipuncture attempts). The most favourable outcomes associated with real-time US guidance were found in studies of inexperienced operators.

Potential for Harm

The additional equipment and manipulation associated with real-time US guidance for CVC insertion may increase the rate of catheter-related infections, but published studies have not included these complications. In emergency settings, the increased length of time required to place CVCs under US guidance (usually an additional 30 seconds to several minutes) may result in unacceptable delays. Potential harmful consequences resulting from real-time US guidance for CVC placement relate to changes in training and subsequent dependence on this technology. Supporters of this technology argue that increased competence and anatomic knowledge gained with US guidance will enhance performance of customary, unaided CVC placement. It is unclear if trainees who have performed CVC placement only with US assistance will have different complication rates when placing CVCs in practice settings without US equipment. Therefore, for certification of qualification, trainees may need to demonstrate competence with both US and non-US guided CVC placement.

Costs and Implementation

The major impediments to the widespread implementation of US guidance for CVC insertion are the purchase costs of the US machines. A typical machine costs $11,000-16,000 (including the probes), with a single machine able to serve most critical care units. Depending on the layout of units placing CVCs, an average 400-bed hospital would require 1-3 machines for use outside of the operating room. (Departments of Anesthesia may require only one or two machines, as experienced anesthesiologists can continue to place most CVCs without US guidance). Hospitals in which nurses place *peripherally inserted central catheter* (PICC) lines using US guidance typically facilitate this function with a single machine, which could be dually used for CVCs depending on workflow and volume. In one study, the price of the Doppler-Smart needles (which are not required for non-Doppler US guidance) was $40-70 as compared with $3-5 for the standard needles. The cost of training new operators (including those whose only prior experience is with the landmark technique) requires further evaluation.

Comment

Real-time US guidance for CVC insertion, with or without Doppler assistance, improves catheter insertion success rates, reduces the number of venipuncture attempts prior to successful placement, and reduces the number of complications associated with catheter insertion. However, these benefits may not accrue until after the initial learning period for operators already experienced in the landmark techniques. There are no studies comparing the impact of CVC insertion with US guidance on overall patient outcomes (e.g., mortality, length of stay). In addition, many of the complications associated with CVC insertion are minor or easily treated. The reduction in venipuncture attempts is likely associated with reductions in the pain and discomfort associated with CVC placement, though this has not been measured.

The greatest benefit of US guidance may apply to the novice or inexperienced operator and for all operators in high-risk situations. Patients with one or more risk factors, (e.g., critically ill patients on positive pressure ventilation with generalized edema and coagulopathy), may reap the greatest benefit. CVC insertion training incorporating real-time ultrasound guided techniques may provide additional valuable learning benefits for new operators. This knowledge may improve the success rate of insertion of CVCs without US guidance. Simulation training has demonstrated improved identification of the desired veins with US as compared to landmark techniques.

Finally, it should be noted that in addition to real-time US guidance, other approaches may reduce the risks associated with CVC insertion. PICC lines are gaining widespread acceptance and may be an acceptable substitute for CVCs for certain indications (e.g., long-term IV access or parenteral nutrition). US guidance has also been demonstrated to improve the insertion of PICCs. Increases in the use of PICCs may help justify the purchase of ultrasound machines by individual hospitals.

For patients requiring replacement of existing CVCs, guidewire exchanges offer a way of inserting new catheters without new venipuncture attempts. A systematic review has found that guidewire exchanges are associated with fewer mechanical complications than new-site replacement, but may be associated with greater risks for catheter-related infections.

Alternative methods for teaching CVC insertion skills to novices (e.g., first-year resident physicians and medical students) have successfully employed multidisciplinary approaches including cadaver demonstrations. Future methods for teaching CVC insertion may employ computerized technologies for simultions . Haptic, or touch-related techniques use virtual reality models to create immersive simulated environments that recreate the sensation of performing a procedure. Through the use of this and other new technologies, novice operators may gain experience and confidence prior to clinical CVC insertion attempts and further improve patient safety.

PRE-ANESTHESIA CHECKLISTS TO I MPROVE PATIENT SAFETY

No matter how rote the task or how vigilant the anesthesiologist, “slips” and other errors represent expected aspects of human performance. Evaluation and subsequent improvement of standard checkout procedures promises to increase patient safety in the perioperative period by removing more of the "human factors" so often implicated in anesthesia adverse events. The use of pre-flight checklists has been considered a key method in improving airline safety, largely due to the regular systematizing of complex procedures, and improvement of team dynamics through authority-neutral tasks. A checklist system has been proposed as part of routine pre-anesthesia care, with the American Society of Anesthesiologists and the US Food and Drug Administration (FDA) issuing general guidelines supporting checklists in 1986. Subsequently, anesthesia professional societies in Great Britain and Europe adopted similar standards.

Practice Description

In 1987, the FDA published the "Anesthesia Apparatus Checkout Recommendations" in the *Federal Register* (February, 1987). This "checkout list" provides practitioners with a standardized approach to checking anesthetic equipment prior to its use in order to ensure that the delivery system is correctly connected, adjusted, and functional. The original checklist included 24 specific processes to be performed as an initial checkout at the beginning of each day; 11 are performed between cases and after initial equipment evaluation. Many clinicians regarded these protocols as too long and complex for routine use. Parties involved in revising the recommendations agreed that the average clinician should be able to check an anesthesia machine in 5 minutes or less (not possible with the 1987 recommendations). The revised checklist included only 14 major processes, 9 of which can be omitted or substantially abbreviated when the anesthesia provider uses the same equipment in successive cases. The revised recommendations are available online.

Prevalence and Severity of the Target Safety Problem

The earliest observational studies of mishaps within anesthesia found that equipment failure was the cause of 14% of anesthesia critical incidents. Subsequent studies reduced this estimate considerably. Although equipment failure is now implicated in only 4% of anesthesia adverse events, 22% are related to failing to check equipment adequately. Equipment failures can result in delivery of hypoxic gas mixtures or excessive doses of inhalational agent, or hypoventilation due to ventilator failure. These situations can be catastrophic if unrecognized, and even if recognized may result in significant morbidity (e.g., delayed extubation, stroke, or myocardial infarction).

Opportunities for Impact

The FDA checkout list is considered a template which local users are "encouraged to modify to accommodate differences in equipment and variations in local clinical practice." Estimating the frequency with which it or other checklists are used (in modified or unmodified forms) in anesthesia practice would be speculative, but a survey of 4 states suggests that usage is minimal. There are 41.5 million inpatient procedures each year requiring anesthesia in the US. Probably about half of these involve general anesthesia. Therefore, although the frequency of equipment failure is low, any improvement in safety from anesthesia preoperative checklists could have substantial impact.

Study Designs

Using a structured MEDLINE search, we identified 15 articles that discussed anesthesia checklists. Of these, only 2 studies came close to meeting our inclusion criteria. Because no other studies could be found, we abstracted these studies and review them here.

The first investigation evaluated the ability of participating providers to detect standardized equipment faults using their own checking methods compared with the FDA checkout list. Although the study involved a prospective design, it does not fit neatly into our classification system because the participants (anesthesiology residents and practitioners) served as their own controls. The second study involved the revised FDA checkout list, and its design was modeled on the previous study.

Study Outcomes

The first study's outcome of interest was the detection of 4 standardized equipment faults created by the investigators (Level 2). The second study used similarly designed outcomes (simulated equipment faults), but defined detection of at least 50% of these faults as the primary outcome (Level 2). Neither study directly connected the use of pre-anesthesia checklists to patient outcomes, although inadequate preanesthesia equipment checks have been implicated in adverse events related to equipment failures, as discussed above.

Evidence for Effectiveness of the Practice

March et al found that the FDA checklist was more likely to detect faults with the nitrous oxide system (65% vs. 43%, $p<0.001$), but that the FDA checklist was no better than individual practitioners' checklists in detecting the 7 other pre-set faults. No method detected 100% of faults, but those physicians with more clinical practice and those with better knowledge of the FDA checklist were more effective at detecting equipment faults. In the study of the revised FDA checklist, approximately half of the participants failed to detect at least half of the faults using both their own methods and the FDA checkout list (no statistically significant difference).

Both of these studies contain important methodologic flaws. The participants knew they were involved in a study assessing their ability to detect machine faults, and so undoubtedly approached this task with increased sensitivity. Moreover, the participants' own methods may have been quite similar to the use of the FDA checklist. Both of these problems bias these studies against finding a difference between checklist and controls. Importantly though, all methods performed poorly in both studies. Thus, even if the FDA checkout list is in fact superior to anesthesia providers' own methods, the observed utility of this practice still is likely to be quite low.

Potential for Harm

We were unable to find literature that implicated checklists as causes of adverse events. There exists a theoretical possibility of delays due to complex checklists, but these have not been borne out in any published studies. There has also been concern raised about compulsory checklist procedures as an unnecessary duplication of work already performed by operating room technical personnel.

Costs and Implementation

The FDA checklist, or local variants thereof, is widely implemented and inexpensive. Although several authors have mentioned that checkout processes are not used in 100% of cases, this does not seem to reflect problems with checklists themselves. The work of March and Crowley suggests that checklists training may be critically important. However, the most important barrier to implementation is the heterogeneity of anesthesia delivery devices themselves, which makes creation of a single, effective, broadly generalizable checklist difficult if not impossible.

Comment

Given its face validity and the theoretical connection

between anesthesia checklists and those used so effectively in aviation, preanesthesia checklists represent plausible safety tools. However, the reliability of modern anesthesia machines has reduced the frequency of mechanical failure to such a degree that adverse outcomes due to anesthesia machine failure are exceedingly rare. The checklists examined in the cited studies only examine the integrity of the anesthesia machine and ventilatory monitors, not cardiovascular monitors, airway equipment, intravenous apparatus, infusion pumps, or medications. Standardized checklists for these other critical components of anesthesia care do not exist in the literature. This may explain the paucity of literature exploring the use of checklists and their real effects on patient outcomes.

Furthermore, the inability of anesthesiologists to detect preset faults in the cited studies may simply reflect the infrequency with which such faults are encountered in modern anesthesia practice. The face validity of checklists and the difficulty of "probing" their value in clinical studies make additional "proof of concept" studies unlikely. Although future investigations could not ethically study the anesthesia machine checklist *per se*, they could seek to determine more effective methods for its implementation, or could develop additional checklists with a broader scope.

The little evidence we have been able to uncover suggests that, like the use of voluntary guidelines elsewhere in medicine, checklists are not used uniformly. This may result from a sense that these checks are low-yield, redundant, onerous, or all of the above.

The need for effective checkout procedures is likely to grow as the complexity of anesthesia equipment increases. This will increase the need to make checklists more sensitive and specific in detecting faults, while improving usability.

These worthy goals may then serve as templates for other technologically dependent medical specialties, such as cardiac electrophysiology, and interventional radiology.

THE IMPACT OF INTRAOPERATIVE MONITORING ON PATIENT SAFETY

Until the 1960s, intraoperative monitoring consisted of a blood pressure cuff, electrocardiogram (ECG), stethoscope, and the vigilance of the anesthesiologist. Over the next 2 decades, the array of available monitors burgeoned, and clinical practice varied widely. In 1986, in an effort to improve patient safety, standards for intraoperative monitoring were developed and implemented by the American Society of Anesthesiologists (ASA). They have been almost universally adopted by anesthesia providers in the United States and now form the standard of care in this country. Concurrently with the implementation of better monitoring, anesthesia-related mortality has fallen sharply. Proponents of monitoring claim that better monitoring is the reason for improvement in patient safety. Others have claimed that advances in knowledge and training combined with the development of safer medications have had as much impact on patient safety as the adoption of monitoring standards. In this chapter, we evaluate the evidence linking intraoperative monitoring to patient safety.

Practice Description

Intraoperative monitoring involves the use of mechanical devices to record and display physiologic parameters such as heart rate, blood pressure, oxygen saturation, and temperature. Standard routine monitoring is noninvasive, employing blood pressure cuff, ECG, and pulse oximetry. Invasive monitors such as arterial and central venous catheters and transesophageal echocardiography may provide more detailed and timely physiologic information, but also pose an increased risk for iatrogenic complications. In practice these monitors are used selectively, and are not reviewed here.

Prevalence and Severity of the Target Safety Problem

Death due to anesthesia has become rare. In one large Canadian study involving 27,184 inpatients who underwent anesthesia, physician review of 115 randomly selected "major events" classified less than 20% as having any anesthetic involvement, with no deaths even partially attributed to anesthesia. In the United States, the mortality due to general anesthesia has been estimated at approximately 5000 deaths per year (in the 1970s), with approximately half that number estimated in the 1980s. Thus, general anesthesia represents the one aspect of healthcare where the risk of death is low enough to rival the safety record achieved in other high-risk industries such as aviation.

By contrast, morbid events (complications) related to anesthetic care are likely more prevalent and difficult to classify as preventable or unavoidable. Because certain aspects of monitoring may reduce the incidence of morbid events unrelated to anesthesia, assessing the impact of monitoring practices solely on anesthetic outcomes may be inappropriate. For example, detection of a consistent decrease in intraoperative blood pressure may signal unrecognized bleeding, allowing the anesthesiologist to alert the surgeon to this possibility and prompting appropriate management. While intraoperative hemorrhage does not represent an anesthetic complication, intraoperative blood pressure monitoring can clearly contribute to the overall safety of the surgical patient. Thus, the scope of intraoperative morbidity targeted by anesthetic monitoring practices is much broader than the set of possible complications attributable solely to the administration of anesthesia.

Opportunities for Impact

In the United States, there are no mandatory regulations for monitoring practices. However, virtually all anesthesiologists abide by the monitoring standards set forth by the 1986 ASA standards, last modified in 1998. Although these standards were implemented with only speculative evidence of their benefit, few clinicians doubt their merit.

Study Designs

Using a structured MEDLINE search, we identified articles presenting data related to the impact of perioperative monitoring. Many of these studies involved Level 4 designs (e.g., observational studies without a control group). For instance, several of the articles reported data from the Australian Incident Monitoring Study and involved analysis of a case series of 2000 incident reports without accompanying controls. Other studies only indirectly pertained to intraoperative monitoring. One study surveyed anesthesiologists regarding their views on the appropriate alarm settings for intraoperative blood pressure monitoring. Another focused on the personnel performing intraoperative monitoring—physician anesthesiologists versus certified nurse anesthetists. We chose not to purse this contentious and intensely political comparison, as few studies have compared the outcomes achieved by these two groups. Moreover, our reviewer team did not include a nurse anesthetist, making any conclusions drawn more susceptible to bias. Of the 3 remaining studies, one involved a non-randomized clinical trial (Level 2), but a Level 3 outcome.

The remaining 2 studies met our inclusion criteria. One was a retrospective analysis of anesthesia accidents before and after the implementation of monitoring standards (Level 3), and the other used a prospective, randomized, controlled trial design (Level 1) to assess the impact of pulse oximetry on postoperative complications (Level 1 outcome).

Study Outcomes

The 2 studies meeting the methodologic inclusion criterion reported morbidity and mortality (Level 1) attributable to anesthesia, i.e., a major complication or death occurring in the immediate postoperative period not obviously explained by the patient's underlying condition or the operation itself.

Evidence for Effectiveness of the Practice

Through a review of cases reported to a liability insurer, Eichhorn identified 11 major intraoperative accidents solely attributable to anesthesia among over 1,000,000 cases performed at the nine Harvard hospitals from 1976-1988. Eight of these accidents were judged to be preventable as they were caused by failure to ventilate or to deliver adequate oxygen to the patient. Only one of these accidents occurred after the adoption of monitoring standards in mid-1985, supporting the safety benefit of intraoperative monitoring standards, although the difference in accident frequency was not statistically significant. In a multicenter, randomized, controlled trial of 20,802 surgical patients, Moller et al studied the impact of perioperative pulse oximetry on patient outcome. Despite the large sample, the authors were unable to show a difference in in-hospital mortality or postoperative complications. During anesthesia and in the post-anesthesia care unit (PACU), more episodes of hypoxemia and myocardial ischemia were detected in patients monitored with pulse oximetry.

Potential for Harm

Routine noninvasive monitoring carries minimal

(although not zero) additional risk for iatrogenic complications from the devices themselves. Current standard of practice requires that they be used in all cases of general or regional anesthesia. However the number of monitors and their concomitant alarms raises the possibility of additional harm. A study of monitor alarms in the intensive care unit (ICU) suggested that monitor alarms might actually reduce quality of care because of their high frequency and low specificity. In this study, an alarm occurred every 37 minutes, and in the majority of cases (72%) no change in management was indicated as a result.

Costs and Implementation

The costs of intraoperative monitors are largely fixed in the acquisition cost of the monitoring device. Incremental patient costs for disposables are minimal.

Comment

The inability of a very large multicenter study to detect a benefit in morbidity and mortality from pulse oximetry—by all accounts the most useful monitor—suggests that the magnitude of benefit may be so small that an adequate study to detect this difference may not be feasible. Along with capnography (carbon dioxide monitoring), pulse oximetry is often cited as the monitoring method most able to detect potential critical incidents early enough to prevent adverse outcomes. This conjecture is supported by the ASA Closed Claims Study. Analysing 1175 claims, the study concluded that the combination of pulse oximetry and capnography "could be expected" to help prevent anesthetic-related morbidity and mortality.

Despite a lack of randomized trial data, the practice of noninvasive intraoperative monitoring has become standard of care. This has resulted from the ASA Monitoring Standards and physicians' faith in the practice based on its face value, along with some confirmatory evidence drawn from incident reporting systems. As such, it seems likely that future research into intraoperative monitoring will be unable to study approaches that do not include standard, noninvasive monitoring. Future investigation might seek to determine which monitoring methods detect "near misses" more effectively.

Moving beyond non-invasive techniques, there is a great need to identify which specialized monitors provide a safety benefit in selected patient populations. The use of pulmonary artery catheters for monitoring critically ill patients represents a well-known example of a practice with substantial face validity but unclear impact on patient outcomes. In addition, new, noninvasive alternatives to invasive monitors (e.g., esophageal or spirometry-based cardiac output monitors) may ultimately allow us to obtain the same information at less risk to the patient.

PREVENTION OF CLINICALLY SIGNIFICANT GASTROINTESTINAL BLEEDING IN INTENSIVE CARE UNIT PATIENTS

Stress-related gastric ulceration was first described in the early 1970s, and has since received extensive study. Appreciation of the physiologic changes that promote stress-related gastritis and general improvements in the care of critically ill patients have likely played a role in reducing the frequency of this complication. Nonetheless, the use of specific pharmacologic agents for the prevention of stress-related gastrointestinal (GI) bleeding is increasingly promoted as standard therapy in the ICU setting. Despite the common use of these agents, controversy about the evidence supporting this practice remains. Because specific pharmacologic prophylaxis for stress ulceration may increase the risk of other complications (e.g., nosocomial pneumonia) and is associated with significant costs, recent efforts have focused on delineating an appropriate definition of clinically important GI bleeding and identifying patients who derive a clear benefit from pharmacologic prevention of this complication.

Practice Description

This chapter reviews evidence supporting the use of pharmacologic therapies for stress ulcer and GI bleeding prophylaxis in the ICU setting. We considered the use of histamine-2 receptor blocking agents (H2-receptor antagonists) and sucralfate, a mucosal protecting agent. Although the efficacy of aluminum- and magnesium-based antacids has been demonstrated, their use is limited by dosing frequency and side effects. Proton-pump inhibitors (PPIs) and enteral nutrition have also shown benefit in small studies, but there are yet no large randomized evaluations.

Prevalence and Severity of the Target Safety Problem

The risk of stress ulceration and subsequent GI bleeding depends on a patient's underlying illness, its severity, and related comorbidities. Using liberal criteria for assessment of bleeding, early reports estimated the incidence of GI bleeding due to stress ulceration in ICU patients to be as high as 5-25%. However, more recent prospective studies, using stricter definitions of clinically significant GI bleeding and following large cohorts of patients, have revealed more modest estimates of 0.1% in low-risk ICU patients and 2.8% in ventilated patients.

Opportunities for Impact

A recent, prospectively collected database of over 7000 patients admitted to surgical and medical intensive care units at a tertiary care center (1988-95) revealed that 59.9% of patients received pharmacologic prophylaxis with ranitidine or sucralfate for stress ulceration. Another study assessed the annual change in stress ulcer prophylaxis in nearly 3000 patients admitted to a medical intensive care unit at a tertiary care hospital from 1993 to 1996. It found a significant decrease in rates of prophylaxis, with a 71% rate in 1993 progressively decreasing to a 21% rate in 1996, likely reflecting emerging evidence regarding high and low-risk populations in the literature during that time. Identifying appropriate patients for stress ulcer prophylaxis and avoiding its use in other cases both offer potential opportunities for improving patient safety in the ICU.

Study Designs

Although multiple meta-analyses have reviewed the prophylaxis of GI bleeding in critically ill patients, many were performed more than a decade ago. Since then, results of additional randomized trials have been published. More recent, well-designed search strategies, strict quality-scoring of literature, and rigorous adherence to criteria defining clinically significant GI bleeding have improved the breadth and quality of literature captured, likely making older systematic reviews less relevant. Because of these changes in quality measures as well as overlap of information and trials from older reviews contained within more recent ones, only those meta-analyses published within the last 5 years (and large randomized controlled trials not included in these reviews) are included here. A 1996 meta-analysis found 269 studies through a broad search of multiple databases and extensive efforts to find unpublished trials. Sixty-three of these met inclusion criteria. The analysis evaluated multiple types of prophylaxis for GI bleeding, including antacids, H2-antagonists, and sucralfate. The study authors compared each type of prophylaxis to placebo and to each other when literature was available. The same study group then followed-up unanswered questions from their meta-analysis with a large randomized controlled trial (RCT) of 1200 patients, comparing ranitidine to sucralfate without a placebo group.

A more recent meta-analysis abstracted evidence from the literature to compare ranitidine (instead of all H2-antagonists) versus placebo, and sucralfate versus placebo for GI bleed prophylaxis in the ICU. The search methods were less rigorous and the target population narrower than the 1996 meta-analysis, but the authors claimed to assess a more clinically relevant population and outcome. Results from 2 prospective cohort studies that evaluated risk factors for occurrence of clinically important GI bleeding also provide key recommendations regarding clinical practice.

Study Outcomes

Both meta-analyses and the large RCT reported outcomes of clinically important GI bleeding and nosocomial pneumonia (Level 1). The 1996 meta-analysis and randomized trial also evaluated overt GI bleeding and mortality. Cohort studies (Level 2) present results of multivariate regression analyses, identifying the salient risk factors for clinically important GI bleeding in the ICU patient.

Evidence for Effectiveness of the Practice

The outcomes for the 2 meta-analyses and large RCT. The disparity in results of the meta-analyses is partly due to differing article selection criteria. While the 1996 analysis evaluated all H2-antagonists, the 2000 study excluded trials evaluating cimetidine because of its virtual replacement (attributable to its undesirable side effect profile) by ranitidine in current clinical practice. Excluding studies with cimetidine substantially reduced the number of studies available for review. Additionally, the 1996 study evaluated comparisons of therapies to each other as well as to placebo, while the

2000 study only considered trials of effectiveness with a placebo control as relevant.

The 2000 meta-analysis found no statistically significant reduction in clinically important GI bleeding when comparing H2-antagonist agents with placebo, or sucralfate to placebo. However, the 1996 study revealed a significant difference between ranitidine and placebo for clinically important GI bleeding. It was unable to demonstrate such a difference between ranitidine and sucralfate. The results of these 2 reviews reveal discrepant findings, in large part due to exclusion of cimetidine in the 2000 study. However, that study also included at least one moderate-sized trial that used remarkably strict criteria for defining clinically important GI bleeding. This factor likely contributed an element of bias towards the null result in that meta-analysis.

Furthermore, the large RCT (1998) comparing ranitidine to sucralfate, without a placebo comparison group, revealed a statistically significant difference in the rate of clinically important upper GI bleeding, favouring H2-antagonists. In this RCT the number needed to treat (NNT) with ranitidine compared to placebo to prevent one clinically important GI bleed compared to placebo was 47. However, no reduction in mortality or length of ICU stay was found. Interpretation of the results of the RCT are complicated by: 1) wide confidence intervals surrounding the relative risk estimate; 2) very small numbers of patients with clinically important GI bleeding (ranitidine group: 10/596; sucralfate group: 23/604), only 42% of whom had endoscopic confirmation of the source of bleed; 3) a large number of patients (70%) receiving concomitant enteral nutrition, believed to reduce the risk of GI bleeding unreported incidence of coagulopathy or duration of prophylaxis prior to GI bleeding.

The 2 large cohort studies found respiratory failure (odds ratio 15.6, $p<0.001$), coagulopathy (odds ratio 4.3, $p<0.001$), and renal insufficiency (relative risk 1.16, $p=0.023$) to be independent risk factors for predicting clinically important GI bleeding in ICU patients. Enteral nutrition had a protective effect on GI bleed outcome (relative risk 0.30, $p=0.004$). Even though previous studies found a high incidence of overt GI bleeding among head trauma patients, this was not supported by the most recent cohort study cited above, which evaluated ventilated head trauma patients.

Potential for Harm

The harm evaluated in the 2 recent meta-analyses and large RCT. All 3 studies showed either a trend toward reduction or statistically significant reduction of nosocomial pneumonia in sucralfate groups compared with ranitidine groups. The number needed to harm (NNH) to cause one nosocomial pneumonia with ranitidine compared with sucralfate was calculated as 21 to 34. However, this effect was not statistically significant in the RCT. No study demonstrated a harmful effect for ranitidine compared to placebo.

Costs and Implementation

One cost-effectiveness analysis extracted relevant literature from MEDLINE between 1985 and 1995, representing 15 controlled clinical trials (Level 1). Assumptions made in the analysis included equal efficacy for the H2-antagonist cimetidine and sucralfate, a baseline risk of bleeding of 6%, and a 50% risk-reduction due to prophylaxis. The average cost per bleeding episode averted was $1144 for sucralfate, but 6.5 times greater for cimetidine. However, low-risk patients amassed a cost per bleeding episode averted of $103,725 compared to a cost of $279 for very high-risk patients. Cost per bleeding episode averted increased significantly if the risk of nosocomial pneumonia was included in the analysis. The large RCT reported no difference in the duration of ICU stay for the group treated with ranitidine compared with the group treated with sucralfate (9 days for each group). However, no placebo group was used.

Comment

Overall, the evidence available in the literature does not conclusively demonstrate that the benefits of GI prophylaxis outweigh its risks for every patient admitted to the intensive care unit. As refinements have been made in defining *clinically* important and significant episodes of GI bleeding, the population that may reap benefit from prophylaxis has narrowed substantially. In turn, a reduction in the use of prophylactic agents has followed. Most recent estimates reveal a negligible incidence of clinically important stress-related GI bleeding in low-risk ICU patients (approximately 0.1%) and a small incidence (less than 3%) in higher-risk patients. Improvements in overall ICU care and use of enteral nutrition may be contributing to this decrease in incidence.

Although a statistical benefit of H2-antagonists compared with placebo or with sucralfate has been shown in some studies, the overall *clinical* benefit of these agents has been disputed. Some research shows a greater absolute number of nosocomial pneumonia cases related to therapy with H2-antagonists than the benefit from reduction in GI bleeding, causing the NNH to be potentially smaller than the NNT. Furthermore, the overall cost-to-benefit ratio of prophylaxis increases dramatically in lower-risk patients, as shown in the analysis noted above that accounted for increases in nosocomial pneumonia. Thus, the clear benefit of administering H2-antagonists to prevent GI bleeding among many patients in an ICU remains to be shown. This is partly due to variations in the definition of clinically significant bleeding and pneumonia. Additional large trials are necessary to identify the patients who truly derive net benefit from this practice, as published evidence does not yet support this practice for many patients currently receiving the therapy. At the present time, clinicians may consider use of prophylactic agents, an H2-antagonist or sucralfate, to prevent clinically important GI bleeding in very high-risk patients admitted to the ICU. Such patients may include those with respiratory failure, coagulopathy, renal failure, and/or burns (the latter group has been excluded from most studies because its risk is believed to be so great). However, the risk of pneumonia may influence clinicians to use prophylactic agents only in patients with multiple risk factors for GI bleeding, and simply provide enteral nutrition to others at less risk. The use of PPIs requires further study before any recommendation can be made regarding them. Further research should focus on identifying subgroups of patients who do derive net benefit from ranitidine or other acid-reducing agents.

PROTOCOLS FOR HIGH-RISK DRUGS: REDUCING ADVERSE DRUG EVENTS RELATED TO ANTICOAGULANTS

Published studies of adverse drug events and multiple case reports have consistently identified certain classes of medications as particularly serious threats to patient safety. These "high risk" medications include concentrated electrolyte solutions such as potassium chloride, intravenous insulin, chemotherapeutic agents, intravenous opiate analgesics, and anticoagulants such as heparin and warfarin. Analyses of some of the adverse events involving these mediations have led to important recommendations regarding their administration. Examples include the use of order templates for chemotherapeutic agents, removal of intravenous electrolyte solutions from general ward stock, and protocols for reviewing the settings of intravenous pumps delivering continuous or frequent doses of opiates. While these recommendations have high face validity, they have generally not been subject to formal evaluation regarding their impact in reducing the targeted adverse events. By contrast, several practices relating to the management of patients receiving anticoagulants have been evaluated quite extensively, and therefore constitute the focus of this chapter.

Heparin and warfarin are medications whose use or misuse carry significant potential for injury. Subtherapeutic levels can lead to thromboembolic complications in patients with atrial fibrillation or deep venous thrombosis (DVT), while supratherapeutic levels can lead to bleeding complications. These medications are commonly involved in ADEs for a variety of reasons, including the complexity of dosing and monitoring, patient compliance, numerous drug interactions, and dietary interactions that can affect drug levels. Strategies to improve both the dosing and monitoring of these high-risk drugs have potential to reduce the associated risks of bleeding or thromboembolic events.

Practice Description

The practices reviewed in this chapter are all intended to reduce dosing and/or monitoring errors for heparin and warfarin, as follows:

— *Heparin dosing protocols ("nomograms")* typically involve a standard initial bolus and infusion rate, instructions for when to draw the first partial thromboplastin time (PTT), and orders for dosing adjustments in response to this and subsequent values (so nurses can adjust doses automatically). In some cases, the initial bolus and infusion rates are based on patient weight.

— *Inpatient anticoagulation services* for both heparin and warfarin (with or without dosing nomograms) typically consist of pharmacist-run services that provide daily pharmacy input on dosing and monitoring for patients on heparin and/or warfarin (We excluded studies focusing solely on warfarin prophylaxis in orthopedic patients).

— *Outpatient anticoagulation clinics* provide coordinated services for managing outpatient warfarin therapy. Services typically include anticoagulation monitoring and follow-up, warfarin dose adjustment, and patient education. These clinics are usually run by pharmacists or nurses operating with physician back-up, and sometimes following specific dosing nomograms.

— *Patient self-monitoring* using a home finger-stick device and self-adjustment of warfarin dosages using a nomogram (The accuracy of these devices and the comparability of patients' and professional readings have been extensively evaluated).

Prevalence and Severity of the Target Safety Problem

Intravenous heparin and oral warfarin are commonly used medications for cardiac disease and thromboembolism in the inpatient and outpatient settings. While in the aggregate they are highly beneficial, these drugs can have significant morbidities unless they are dosed and monitored appropriately. For example, inadequate therapeutic dosing of heparin can lead to increased length of stay and the potential for clot formation and/or propagation. The risk of recurrent thromboembolism is reduced if the therapeutic effect of heparin is achieved quickly. In addition, Landefeld et al showed that the frequency of fatal, major, and minor bleeding during heparin therapy was twice that expected without heparin therapy. The effect with warfarin therapy was even more pronounced—approximately 5 times that expected without warfarin therapy. Consistent with this finding, anticoagulants accounted for 4% of preventable ADEs and 10% of potential ADEs in one large inpatient study. Finally, careful drug monitoring in hospitals can reduce ADEs, suggesting that some events are due to inadequate monitoring of therapies and doses. These studies highlight the clear need for safety-related interventions with respect to both the dosing and monitoring of these high-risk drugs in order to prevent thromboembolic and bleeding complications.

Opportunities for Impact

The number of hospitals using weight-based heparin nomograms, or that have established anticoagulation clinics or services is unknown. Although common in some European countries, patient self-management of long-term anticoagulation with warfarin is unusual in the United States as many payers, including Medicare, do not currently cover the home testing technology.

Study Designs

Heparin nomograms were evaluated in one randomized controlled trial (Level 1), one prospective cohort comparison (Level 2) and 4 controlled observational studies (Level 3). Two of these studies involved weight-based nomograms. A third study involving a weight-based nomogram was included with the studies of anticoagulation services, as clinical pharmacists actively managed the dosing protocol. We excluded one retrospective before-after analysis of a weight-based heparin protocol for cardiac intensive care patients, because the method of selecting charts for review was never stated. Moreover, when the authors found an increase in the number of patients with excessive anticoagulation in the intervention group, they chose a second group of control patients (again with an unspecified selection method) for review, and in the end concluded that the difference was not significant. All studies of *outpatient anticoagulation clinics* have been Level 3 studies, typically retrospective before-after analyses, although one study might more appropriately be regarded as a case-control study. A comprehensive review of the literature on various forms of anticoagulation management did not meet the criteria for a systematic review, but referenced all of the additional studies of anticoagulation clinics that we could identify and used quantitative methods to pool their results.

Two studies evaluated the impact of a coordinated *inpatient anticoagulation service* (with or without nomograms for dosing).

Patient self-management of warfarin therapy has been evaluated in at least 3 randomized controlled trials (Level 1) and one non-randomized clinical trial. Because a number of higher-level studies exist, we did not include retrospective cohort analyses (Level 3) addressing this topic.

Study Outcomes

Most studies did not evaluate bleeding complications or had insufficient numbers of patients to evaluate this outcome adequately. One recent study of an anticoagulation clinic's adverse events focused on anticoagulation as the primary outcome (Level 1), as did the review that pooled results from 6 observational studies of anticoagulation clinics. The rest of the studies reported Level 2 outcomes, consisting of various indicators of time to therapeutic anticoagulation and intensity or appropriateness of anticoagulation.

Evidence for Effectiveness of the Practice

— *Heparin nomograms*: As shown in this study, all studies showed a significant decrease (i.e., improvement) in time to achievement of a therapeutic PTT and/or an increase in the proportion of patients in the therapeutic range.

— *Inpatient anticoagulation services*: As shown in this study, both Level 3 studies evaluating this practice showed significant improvements in relevant measures of anticoagulation.

— *Outpatient anticoagulation services for warfarin* (with and without dosing nomograms): the multiple Level 3 studies of this practice showed improvements in relevant measures of anticoagulation, with one exception. This study took place in a semi-rural region of England, and the hospital-based anticoagulation clinic was staffed mainly by junior physician trainees rotating through the clinic. The one study that focused primarily on Level 1 outcomes showed significant reductions in adverse events related to under- or over-anticoagulation.

— *Patient self-management*: Patient self-management achieved superior measures of anticoagulation on one Level 1 comparison with routine care. More impressive is that two Level 1 studies and one Level 2 study reported equivalent or superior measures of anticoagulation for self-management compared with anticoagulation clinics.

Potential for Harm

Heparin nomograms are primarily intended to achieve PTT values within the therapeutic range as quickly as possible. Although none of the studies showed increased bleeding as a result of aggressive anticoagulation, it is important to note that 4 of the 6 studies showed a significant increase in the proportion of patients with PTTs above the target range.

Anticoagulation clinics carry the usual theoretical risk that increased fragmentation of care will introduce new hazards, but no study showed any significant cause for concern.

Patient self-monitoring clearly carries with it risks relating to the possibilities of patient misunderstanding of, or non-compliance with dosing and monitoring protocols. No increases in adverse events were observed in the studies reviewed, but the patients evaluated in these studies, even if randomized, were still chosen from a group of relatively compliant and motivated patients.

Costs and Implementation

For anticoagulation clinics, one study showed reduced costs of $162,058 per 100 patients annually, primarily through reductions in warfarin-related hospitalisations and emergency room visits. Other studies indicate potential cost-savings due to reduced hospitalisations from anticoagulation-related adverse events, or show that the anticoagulation was revenue neutral. Considering without these offsetting potential savings, however, anticoagulant clinics often require institutional subsidy since professional fee or laboratory payments do not fully cover costs. Heparin nomograms may increase lab costs due to more frequent monitoring, but one study calculated that lab costs were offset by the need for fewer heparin boluses.

For patient self-management of warfarin, one study showed that the cost of self-monitoring was $11/international normalized ratio (INR) value and postulated that this would be cost-effective if it reduced the number of clinic visits.

Other studies have suggested that the capillary blood testing devices themselves and the overall practice of patient self-management are cost-effective. In the United States, the home monitoring devices sell for approximately $1000. Factoring in the price of cartridges and assuming the devices operate without requiring repair for 5 years, one source estimated an annual cost of approximately $600.

Implementation of a heparin nonogram appears feasible, and was well received by physicians and nurses. Physician/staff education about the protocols was important to its success. One study showed a high level of physician and patient satisfaction with an anticoagulation clinic. In addition, multiple studies reveal that patients who self-manage warfarin have significantly higher levels of satisfaction and experience less anxiety.

Comment

The primary purpose of heparin nomograms is the timely achievement of therapeutic anticoagulation, and their superiority in this regard (compared with routine care) has been convincingly established. While none of the studies showed adverse consequences of this focus on timely anticoagulation, the trend toward increases in excessive anticoagulation presents safety concerns. Studies powered to detect significant differences in bleeding complications in patients being managed with heparin dosing protocols may be warranted. The literature on anticoagulation clinics consists entirely of observational studies with important possible confounders. Nonetheless, with one exception they are consistently shown to achieve superior measures of anticoagulation, and in one study, superior clinical outcomes.

Among the practices reviewed in this chapter, the literature on patient self-management is perhaps the most impressive. Three randomized trials and one non-randomized clinical trial show that patient control of anticoagulation is at least equivalent, if not superior, to management by usual care or an anticoagulation clinic. Additional observational studies reach the same results. Thus, a relatively substantial literature supports patient self-management for outpatient warfarin therapy for motivated patients able to comply with the monitoring and dosing protocols. These studies clearly involved select groups of patients, so that a larger randomized trial with intention-to-treat analysis would be helpful.

Many insurance carriers in the United States, including Medicare, do not currently subsidize the home testing technology or provide only partial coverage. Despite the relatively high cost of the home testing devices, this practice may nonetheless be cost-effective due to reduced use of other clinical services. A larger US study or detailed cost-effectiveness analysis appears warranted, especially given the higher level of patient satisfaction with this approach as compared with outpatient anticoagulation.

UNIT-DOSE DRUG DISTRIBUTION SYSTEMS

Medication errors are especially likely when health professionals engage in multiple tasks within a short time span. This situation occurs repeatedly in hospitals when pharmacists and technicians load unit-dose carts, and when nurses administer medications. Unit-dose carts are prepared daily, often manually, by technicians and then checked by pharmacists. These carts, containing thousands of patient-specific dosages of drugs, are sent to the wards daily, for nurses to administer medications to patients. Dosing frequencies vary widely, ranging from regular intervals around the clock to "stat" doses given to control acute pain or other symptoms. Medication administration alone is an enormous task for nurses, and one in which they are repeatedly interrupted. It is not surprising that the administration phase of medication use is particularly vulnerable to error. Unit-dose dispensing of medication was developed in the 1960s to support nurses in medication administration and reduce the waste of increasingly expensive medications. Most of the investigations of medication errors and unit-dose dispensing took place from 1970 to 1976. Now, unit-dose dispensing of medications is a standard of practice at hospitals in the United States. This chapter reviews the evidence supporting this practice.

Practice Description

In unit-dose dispensing, medication is dispensed in a package that is ready to administer to the patient. It can be used for medications administered by any route, but oral, parenteral, and respiratory routes are especially common. When unit-dose dispensing first began, hospital pharmacies equipped themselves with machines that packaged and labeled tablets and capsules, one pill per package. They also purchased equipment for packaging liquids in unit-doses. As the popularity of this packaging increased, the pharmaceutical industry began prepackaging pills in unit-of-use form. Many hospitals now purchase prepackaged unit-dose medications. However, it is still common for hospital pharmacies to purchase bulk supplies of tablets and capsules from manufacturers and repackage them in the central pharmacy into unit-dose packages. It is important to note that hospitals vary in the proportion of their wards covered by a unit-dose system.

There are many variations of unit-dose dispensing. As just one example, when physicians write orders for inpatients, these orders are sent to the central pharmacy (by pharmacists, nurses, other personnel, or computer). Pharmacists verify these orders and technicians place drugs in unit-dose carts.

The carts have drawers in which each patient's medications are placed by pharmacy technicians—one drawer for each patient. The drawers are labeled with the patient's name, ward, room, and bed number. Before the carts are transported to the wards, pharmacists check each drawer's medications for accuracy. Sections of each cart containing all medication drawers for an entire nursing unit often slide out and can be inserted into wheeled medication carts used by nurses during their medication administration cycles. A medication administration recording form sits on top of the cart and is used by the nurse to check-off and initial the time of each administration of each medication. The next day, the carts are retrieved from the wards and replaced by a fresh and updated medication supply. Medications that have been returned to the central pharmacy are credited to the patient's account.

A 1999 national survey of drug dispensing and administration practices indicated that three-fourths of responding hospitals had centralized pharmacies, 77% of which were not automated. Larger hospitals and those affiliated with medical schools were more likely to have some component of decentralized pharmacy services. About half of the surveyed hospitals reported drug distribution "systems" that bypassed the pharmacy, including hospitals that reported using floor stocks, borrowing other patients' medications, and hidden drug supplies.

Studies often compare unit-dose dispensing to a *ward stock system*. In this system, nurses order drugs in bulk supplies from the pharmacy; the drugs are stored in a medication room on the ward. Nurses prepare medication cups for each patient during medication administration cycles. The correct number of pills must be taken out of the correct medication container for each cycle and taken to the patient for administration. Liquids must be poured by the nurse from the appropriate bottle and each dose carefully measured. Nurses are responsible for any necessary labeling. Any medications taken from stock bottles and not administered to patients are generally disposed of.

Prevalence and Severity of the Target Safety Problem

The targets of the safety problem for unit-dosing are drug dispensing and administration. Improving these stages probably carries the greatest opportunity to reduce medication errors.

Bates et al identified 530 medical errors in 10,070 written orders for drugs (5.3 errors/100 orders) on 3 medical units observed for 51 days. Of the 530 errors, 5 (0.9%) resulted in an adverse drug event. The most common reason for an error was a missing dose of medication, which occurred in 53% of orders. In a systems analysis of 334 errors causing 264 adverse drug events over 6 months in 2 tertiary care hospitals, 130 errors (39%) resulted from physician ordering, 40 (12%) involved transcription and verification, 38 (11%) reflected problems with pharmacy dispensing, and 126 (38%) were from nursing administration. In other words, 164 (49%) of the errors in the above-cited study were in the dispensing and administration stages. In further research, the investigators found that errors resulting in preventable adverse drug events were more than likely to be those in the administration stage (34%) than those in the dispensing stage (4%) of the medication use process.

Opportunities for Impact

Because unit-dose dispensing now constitutes a standard for approval by the Joint Commission for Accreditation of Healthcare Organisations (JCAHO) and is closely linked to the increasingly common use of automated dispensing devices, there is likely little opportunity for further implementation of this practice in US hospitals. In a 1994 survey of pharmacy directors, 92% of acute care hospitals reported using unit-dose dispensing. Use of unit-dose dispensing is extremely common on general medical and surgical wards, but less so in other locations such as intensive care units, operating rooms, and emergency departments. In these areas, bulk medication stock systems are still found. In a 1999 survey of pharmacy directors, 80% reported that unit-dose dispensing was used for 75% or more of oral doses, and 52% of injectable medications dispensed in their hospitals.

Study Designs

The 5 studies meeting inclusion criteria for this review included 4 Level 3 studies, and one prospectively designed before-after observation (Level 2 design). We excluded the following studies for the reasons outlined:

- Read conducted a study of a unit-dose system applied to respiratory therapy solutions that was focused primarily on measures of efficiency. Volume/concentration errors in preparing respiratory solutions were also discussed, but the method of detection was not stated nor were specific error data provided for the study period.
- Reitberg et al conducted a prospective before-after study with a concurrent comparison floor as a control (Level 2 design) in which medication errors represented the main outcomes (Level 2). During period 1 when both wards used the ward stock system, total errors were 4.7% on the ward that remained on ward stock and 34.2% on the ward that used the modified dispensing system. During period 2, the ward stock system had 5.1% error, while the intervention ward (unit-dose) exhibited a

significantly *increased* 18% error rate. Excluding administration-time errors resulted in error rates of 5.1% (conventional system) and 4.8% (unit-dose), which are not significantly different. The greater number of errors on the modified dispensing ward before and after the intervention were attributed by the authors to factors other than the dispensing systems. Because of this problem, and the fact that this study took place in a skilled nursing facility rather than an acute care hospital, we excluded this study.

— Shultz et al conducted a prospective before-after study (Level 2) involving a somewhat complicated comparison. In the baseline period, approximately 50% of wards used a unit-dose system. During the study period, some wards switched to a unit-dose system in which nurses still administered the medications, while other wards adopted an experimental system, in which pharmacists and pharmacy technicians handled all aspects of the mediation dispensing and administration process. The authors report an error rate of 0.64% for complete unit-dose plus pharmacy technician medication system compared to 5.3% in the more conventional unit-dose system in which nurses continue to administer medications ($p<0.001$ for this comparison). The authors repeated their observations 2 years later, and show a persistent marked reduction in the "complete unit-dose system" compared to the nurse-administered unit-dose system. Unfortunately, nowhere do the authors report the error rate in the baseline period in the wards without a unit-dose system. Thus, none of the results reported by the authors relate specifically to the conversion from a multi-dose to a unit-dose system.

In addition, 2 of the relevant references identified almost certainly reported the same data. The 2 papers have only one author in common, but they come from the same institution, involve study wards of the same size and observation periods of the same duration, and report identical error rates for the main comparison. Lastly, we were unable to obtain one of the original studies of the unit-dose system within the timeline of the project. The data from this study appears to have been published only as a technical report. Other publications related to this study and which we were able to obtain did not provide sufficient detail on the aspects of the study relating to medication errors to permit abstraction or inclusion in this chapter. The published reports of a study conducted in a private hospital similarly did not contain sufficient detail about the study methods or results to permit abstraction and inclusion.

Study Outcomes

Studies reported errors measured by direct observation using a methodology that was first described by Barker. All of these studies involved Level 2 outcomes.

Evidence for Effectiveness of the Practice

Though the practice of unit-dose dispensing is generally well accepted and has been widely implemented, the evidence for its effectiveness is modest. Most of the published studies reported reductions in medication errors of omission and commission with unit-dose dispensing compared with alternative dispensing systems such as ward stock systems. One exception was the international study by Dean, which compared a United States hospital using unit-dose and transcription of medication orders with a United Kingdom hospital using ward stock and no transcription of orders. The results of this study indicated that the United Kingdom hospital had less than half the errors of the United States hospital. The study groups were often difficult to compare because of differing cultures, hospitals, or nursing care units. Moreover, co-interventions undoubtedly confounded the results.

Potential for Harm

Unit-dosing shifts the effort and distraction of medication processing, with its potential for harm, from the nursing ward to central pharmacy. It increases the amount of time nurses have to do other tasks but increases the volume of work within the pharmacy. Like the nursing units, central pharmacies have their own distractions that are often heightened by the unit-dose dispensing process itself, and errors do occur. Overall, unit-dose appears to have little potential for harm. The results of most of the Level 2 observational studies seem to indicate that it is safer than other forms of institutional dispensing. However, the definitive study to determine the extent of harm has not yet been conducted.

A major advantage of unit-dose dispensing is that it brings pharmacists into the medication use process at another point to reduce error. Yet, as pointed out in the Practice Description above, about half of the hospitals in a national survey bypass pharmacy involvement by using floor stock, borrowing patients' medications, and hiding medication supplies.

Costs and Implementation

The cost considerations of unit-dose dispensing are mainly a trade-off between pharmacy and nursing personnel. The pharmacy personnel involved are mainly technicians who load unit-dose ward carts for the pharmacists to check and may package some medications that are commercially unavailable in unit-dose form. The pharmacist must verify that the correct medication and dosage of each medication is sent to the ward for the nurse to administer. Nursing time to maintain a drug inventory is reduced, allowing more time for other nursing activities. A variable cost of unit-dose dispensing is the cost of equipment and supplies to those hospitals that wish to do much of the packaging themselves instead of purchasing medications pre-packaged as unit-doses.

Comment

The studies evaluating the practice of unit-dosing contain important methodologic problems and, although yielding somewhat heterogeneous results, are overall relatively consistent in showing a positive impact on error reduction. In contrast to other practices related to medication use, none of the studies evaluated Level 1 outcomes, such as actual adverse drug events. Nonetheless, unit-dose dispensing or some form of automated dispensing of unit-doses has become ubiquitous in American hospitals and a standard of care in the delivery of pharmacy services. Consequently, it is unlikely that more rigorous studies could now be conducted.

THE RETAINED SURGICAL SPONGE

Although less likely to garner public notoriety, errors relating to the failure to remove surgical instruments at the end of a procedure, (i.e., needles, knife blades, electrosurgical adapters and safety pins) or sponges (known as gossypiboma; *gossypium*: Latin, cotton; *boma*: Swahili, place of concealment) are no less egregious than the better known mishaps such as "wrong-site surgery".

Retained materials may cause an acute foreign body reaction with local or systemic signs that prompt investigation and reoperation. Alternatively, a fibrinous response may be elicited, and the retained instrument or sponge may become apparent some time after the original surgical procedure either serendipitously, or via fistulisation into local structures. The medical literature is scattered with reports of presentations of retained sponges found days, months, or even years after the original surgery. While many cases of retained foreign body do not cause harm, some clearly do. Nevertheless, the Joint Commission on Accreditation for Healthcare Organisation's (JCAHO) sentinel event policy specifically mentions that "unintentionally retained foreign body without major permanent loss of function" do not require reporting. Although JCAHO's decision suggests that it considers these events less egregious than reportable sentinel events (e.g., wrong patient surgery), retained foreign body events are far more common. This chapter reviews the problem and the scanty literature regarding safety practices to reduce the incidence of retained sponges and instruments.

Practice Description

Surgeons and operating room teams rely upon the practice of *sponge, sharp and instrument counts* as a means to eliminate retained surgical instruments. Counts are also a method of infection control and inventory control, and a means to prevent injury from contaminated sharps and instruments. Four separate counts have been recommended: the first when the instruments are set up or the sponges unpackaged, a second before the surgical procedure begins, a third as closure begins, and the final count performed during subcuticular or skin closure. Use of this simple preventative measure is not universal. In fact, the process by which counts are performed is not standardized and is often modified according to individual hospital policy. Even when present, counts are frequently omitted or abbreviated in emergency or transvaginal surgeries, or for vaginal deliveries.An adjunctive procedure to the count, used when the count could delay care and jeopardize patients' lives or when an incorrect count is established, is an x-ray examination to detect radiopaque objects. Since this practice is not routinely used it will not be discussed here.

Prevalence and Severity of the Target Safety Problem

A literature search revealed few data to describe population or even hospital-level information regarding the prevalence of retained surgical materials. One study from a medical malpractice insurance company reported 40 cases in a 7-year period, or about 1% of all claims. Because this estimate is based on malpractice insurance claims, it is sure to be a gross underestimate of the actual incidence. A recent unstructured review cited "a prevalence ranging from 1/100 to 1/5000," and an associated mortality ranging from 11 to 35%, citing non-English language medical references. Other reports are based on case series or descriptions of unusual presentations, as described above. Surgeons may not report these events for a variety of reasons, not the least of which is fear of litigation

Opportunities for Impact

Without accurate prevalence information, the true magnitude of the opportunity for impact is unclear.

Study Designs and Outcomes

Only one study provided even indirect evidence of the effectiveness of sponge and instrument counts. Kaiser et al, using a retrospective review of medical malpractice claims data from a statewide insurer in Massachusetts, reviewed 67 cases where retained sponges or surgical materials were the primary reason for the claim. This study is a case series without any controls (Level 4 design, Level 2 outcomes) which reported only the outcome of retained sponges, rather than the clinical consequences of these errors.

Evidence for Effectiveness of the Practice

The Kaiser et al study reported that 55% of retained sponges were found after abdominal surgery and 16% after vaginal delivery. In cases with retained sponges, sponge counts had been falsely correct in 76% of non-vaginal surgeries; in 10% no sponge count had been performed at all. Falsely correct sponge counts were attributed to team fatigue, difficult operations, sponges "sticking together," or a poor counting system. Incorrect sponge counts that were accepted prior to closure resulted from either surgeons' dismissing the incorrect count without re-exploring the wound, or nursing staff allowing an incorrect count to be accepted. Interestingly, in 3 of 29 cases in which intraoperative x-rays were used to detect radiopaque sponges, the radiograph was falsely negative.

Comment

Although literature describing the incidence of iatrogenic foreign bodies is highly limited in quantity and quality, it is unlikely that these events are as rare as other iatrogenic complications that have drawn considerable national attention. The existing system of sponge and instrument counts probably works well, but we have no evidence to describe its actual failure rate. The little existing evidence suggests that it fails due to human-related factors (i.e., the count is not performed, or is ignored, and that ancillary methods such as x-rays are also fallible. Although some have advocated CT or ultrasonography as additional methods to reduce rates of these adverse events, it is possible that other technologies (e.g., inventory control devices used in retail stores and libraries, possibly including bar coding) may prove to be useful adjuncts. However, there are obvious logistical challenges that make such technologies too impractical at the present time. For now we are left with a paucity of data regarding the prevalence of this error and the effectiveness of preventative measures. Use of anonymous reporting systems may reduce the fear of litigation associated with iatrogenic foreign bodies, and may allow for more accurate assessment of the incidence and causes of these events.

5

Health and Safety Codes: A Case Study

CHAPTER 573 CONTINUING CARE FACILITIES

SUBCHAPTER A. GENERAL PROVISIONS

Sec. 246.001. Short Title

This chapter may be cited as the Texas Continuing Care Facility Disclosure and Rehabilitation Act.

Acts 1989, 71st Leg., ch. 678, Sec. 1, eff. Sept. 1, 1989.

Sec. 246.002. Definitions

In this chapter:

(1) "Board" means the State Board of Insurance.

(2) "Commissioner" means the commissioner of the State Board of Insurance.

(3) "Continuing care" means the furnishing of a living unit, together with personal care services, nursing services, medical services, or other health-related services, regardless of whether the services and the living unit are provided at the same location:

(a) to an individual who is not related by consanguinity or affinity, as determined under Chapter 573, Government Code, to the person furnishing the care; and

(b) under a continuing care contract.

(4) "Continuing care contract" means an agreement that requires the payment of an entrance fee by or on behalf of a resident in exchange for the furnishing of continuing care by a provider and that is effective for:

(a) the life of the resident; or

(b) more than one year.

(5) "Entrance fee" means an initial or deferred transfer of money or other property valued at an amount exceeding three months' rent, made, or promised to be made, as full or partial consideration for acceptance by a provider of a specified individual as a resident. The term does not include a deposit made under a reservation agreement.

(6) "Facility" means a place in which a person provides continuing care to an individual.

(7) "Living unit" means a room, apartment, cottage, or other area that is in a facility and that is set aside for the exclusive use or control of one or more specified individuals.

(8) "Long-term nursing care" means nursing care provided for a period longer than 365 consecutive days.

(9) "Person" means an individual, corporation, association, or partnership, and includes a fraternal or benevolent order or society.

(10) "Provider" means a person who undertakes to provide continuing care in a facility.

(11) "Reservation agreement" means an agreement that requires the payment of a deposit to reserve a living unit for a prospective resident.

(12) "Resident" means an individual entitled to receive continuing care in a facility.

Acts 1989, 71st Leg., ch. 678, Sec. 1, eff. Sept. 1, 1989. Amended by Acts 1991, 72nd Leg., ch. 14, Sec. 95, eff. Sept. 1, 1991; Acts 1991, 72nd Leg., ch. 561, Sec. 31, eff. Aug. 26, 1991; Acts 1993, 73rd Leg., ch. 953, Sec. 1, eff. Sept. 1, 1993; Acts 1995, 74th Leg., ch. 76, Sec. 5.95(27), eff. Sept. 1, 1995.

Sec. 246.003. Board Powers and Duties.

(a) The board shall regulate providers as provided by this chapter.

(b) The board may adopt rules and take other action as necessary to administer and enforce this chapter.

Acts 1989, 71st Leg., ch. 678, Sec. 1, eff. Sept. 1, 1989.

Sec. 246.004. Rights of Residents

A resident receiving care in a portion of a facility licensed to provide nursing home care, personal care, or custodial care is entitled to all statutory rights provided to a nursing home, personal care, or custodial care resident.

Acts 1989, 71st Leg., ch. 678, Sec. 1, eff. Sept. 1, 1989.

Sec. 246.005. Licensing for Certain Tax Purposes

A facility regulated under this chapter is licensed for purposes of Section 151.314, Tax Code.

Acts 1989, 71st Leg., ch. 678, Sec. 1, eff. Sept. 1, 1989.

Sec. 246.006. Quality of Care

The commissioner may not regulate or in any manner inquire into the quality of care provided in a facility.

Acts 1989, 71st Leg., ch. 678, Sec. 1, eff. Sept. 1, 1989.

Sec. 246.007. Reduction of Fees

The commissioner shall reduce the annual filing fees under this chapter if the cumulative amount of the fees exceeds the actual cost of regulation.

Acts 1989, 71st Leg., ch. 678, Sec. 1, eff. Sept. 1, 1989.

SUBCHAPTER B. CERTIFICATE OF AUTHORITY

Sec. 246.021. Certificate of Authority Required

Unless a provider holds a certificate of authority issued under this subchapter, the provider may not:

(1) acquire a facility;

(2) enter into a continuing care contract; or

(3) enter into a reservation agreement unless the agreement provides for the full refund, for any reason, of a deposit paid in connection with the agreement.

Acts 1989, 71st Leg., ch. 678, Sec. 1, eff. Sept. 1, 1989. Amended by Acts 1993, 73rd Leg., ch. 953, Sec. 2, eff. Sept. 1, 1993.

Sec. 246.022. Application for Issuance of Certificate of Authority

(A) The commissioner shall adopt rules stating the information an applicant for a certificate of authority must submit.

(B) On receiving an application for a certificate of authority, the commissioner shall conduct a hearing on the application.

(C) The commissioner shall grant an application for a certificate of authority if the commissioner finds that:

(1) the applicant or the facility is financially sound;

(2) the competence, experience, and integrity of the applicant, its board of directors, its officers, or its management make it in the public interest to issue the certificate; and

(3) the applicant is capable of complying with this chapter.

(D) The commissioner shall issue an order approving or disapproving an application not later than the 180th day after the date on which the application is filed.

(E) The commissioner may limit issuance of certificates of authority to incorporated entities only.

Acts 1989, 71st Leg., ch. 678, Sec. 1, eff. Sept. 1, 1989.

Sec. 246.023. Mandatory Issuance of Certificate of Authority to Certain Facilities

(A) The commissioner shall issue a certificate of authority for a facility that:

(1) was occupied by at least one resident on September 1, 1987;

(2) was under construction on September 1, 1987; or

(3) incurred substantial financial obligations before September 1, 1987, related to the development of the facility.

(B) A certificate of authority issued under this section may be suspended or revoked as any other certificate.

(C) This section prevails over Section 246.022.

Acts 1989, 71st Leg., ch. 678, Sec. 1, eff. Sept. 1, 1989.

Sec. 246.024. Transfer of Certificate of Authority

A certificate of authority may not be transferred without the prior approval of the commissioner.

Acts 1989, 71st Leg., ch. 678, Sec. 1, eff. Sept. 1, 1989. Amended by Acts 1991, 72nd Leg., ch. 14, Sec. 96, eff. Sept. 1, 1991.

Sec. 246.025. Suspension or Revocation of Certificate of Authority

The commissioner may suspend or revoke a provider's certificate of authority if the provider:

(1) draws on its entrance fee escrow in an amount greater than provided for by Section 246.073;

(2) draws on its loan reserve fund escrow in an amount greater than provided for by Section 246.078; or

(3) intentionally violates this chapter.

Acts 1989, 71st Leg., ch. 678, Sec. 1, eff. Sept. 1, 1989. Amended by Acts 1991, 72nd Leg., ch. 14, Sec. 97, eff. Sept. 1, 1991.

Sec. 246.026. Management by Others

A holder of a certificate of authority may not contract for management of the facility unless the commissioner is notified of the contract.

Acts 1989, 71st Leg., ch. 678, Sec. 1, eff. Sept. 1, 1989.

Sec. 246.027. Certificate of Authority Fees

(A) Except as provided by Subsection (b), a facility that files an application for a certificate of authority must pay to the commissioner a fee of $10,000.

(B) A facility that files an application for a certificate of authority issued under Section 246.023 must pay to the commissioner:

(1) a fee of $500; and

(2) a fee of $2 for each living unit in the facility, excluding

a unit devoted to that portion of the facility that is a licensed nursing home.

Acts 1989, 71st Leg., ch. 678, Sec. 1, eff. Sept. 1, 1989.

BCHAPTER C. CONTINUING CARE CONTRACTS AND DISCLOSURE STATEMENTS

Sec. 246.041. Precontractual Recording Requirements

(A) A provider shall file with the board a current disclosure statement that meets the requirements of this subchapter and shall file copies of the agreements establishing the escrows under Subchapter D or a verified statement explaining that an escrow is not required before the provider:

(1) contracts to provide continuing care in a facility located or to be located in this state;

(2) extends the term of an existing continuing care contract in a facility that is located or to be located in this state and that requires or allows an entrance fee from any person, regardless of whether the extended contract requires an entrance fee; or

(3) including a person acting on the provider's behalf, solicits for an individual who is a resident of this state a continuing care contract in this state.

(B)A contract is solicited in this state if, during the 12-month period preceding the date on which a continuing care contract for a facility is signed or accepted by either party, information concerning the facility or the availability of a continuing care contract for the facility is given:

(1) by personal, telephone, mail, or other communication directed to and received by a person at a location in this state; or

(2) in a paid advertisement published or broadcast from

within this state, other than in a publication in which more than two-thirds of the circulation is outside this state.

Acts 1989, 71st Leg., ch. 678, Sec. 1, eff. Sept. 1, 1989.

Sec. 246.042. Delivery Disclosure Statement

(A) A provider who has not been issued a certificate of authority under Subchapter B must deliver a disclosure statement to any person from whom the provider accepts a deposit in connection with a reservation agreement before the provider accepts the deposit.

(B) A provider who has been issued a certificate of authority under Subchapter B must deliver a disclosure statement to a person with whom a continuing care contract is to be made before the earlier of:

(1) the execution of the continuing care contract; or

(2) the transfer of any entrance fee or nonrefundable deposit to the provider by or on behalf of the person.

(C) The most recently filed disclosure statement is the only statement that:

(1) is current for purposes of this chapter; and

(2) may be delivered under this section.

Acts 1989, 71st Leg., ch. 678, Sec. 1, eff. Sept. 1, 1989. Amended by Acts 1993, 73rd Leg., ch. 953, Sec. 3, eff. Sept. 1, 1993.

Sec. 246.043. Cover Page of Disclosure Statement

The cover page of a disclosure statement must state:

(1) the date of the statement in a prominent location and in type that is boldfaced, capitalized, underlined, or otherwise set out from the surrounding written

material so as to be conspicuous;

(2) that if the provider has not been issued a certificate of authority under Subchapter B, this chapter requires the delivery of a disclosure statement to a prospective resident before the payment of any deposit to reserve a living unit;

(3) that this chapter requires the delivery of a disclosure statement to a contracting party before the execution of a continuing care contract or the payment of an entrance fee or nonrefundable deposit; and

(4) that the disclosure statement has not been approved by a governmental agency or representative to ensure the accuracy of its information.

Acts 1989, 71st Leg., ch. 678, Sec. 1, eff. Sept. 1, 1989. Amended by Acts 1991, 72nd Leg., ch. 14, Sec. 98, eff. Sept. 1, 1991; Acts 1993, 73rd Leg., ch. 953, Sec. 4, eff. Sept. 1, 1993.

Sec. 246.044. Contents of Disclosure Statement Provider

(A) The disclosure statement must include the name and business address of the provider and a statement of whether the provider is a partnership, corporation, or other type of legal entity. If the provider is not an individual, the statement must include:

(1) the name and business address of each officer, director, trustee, and managing or general partner; and

(2) the name and business address of each person who has at least a 10 percent interest in the provider and a description of the person's interest in or occupation with the provider.

(B) The provider may include in the disclosure statement

any other material information concerning the facility or the provider.

Acts 1989, 71st Leg., ch. 678, Sec. 1, eff. Sept. 1, 1989.

Sec. 246.045. Contents of Disclosure Statement: Third Party Management

If a person, other than an individual directly employed by the provider, is to be the day-to-day manager of a facility, the disclosure statement must include:

(1) a description of the person's business experience, if any, in the operation or management of a similar facility;

(2) the name and address of any professional service, firm, association, trust, partnership, or corporation that:

(a) has in the person, or in which the person has, at least a 10 percent interest; and

(b) proposes to provide goods, leases, or services to the facility or to the residents of the facility, of an aggregate value of at least $500 in a year;

(3) a description of any goods, leases, or services under Subdivision (2), and a statement of their probable or anticipated cost to the facility, provider, or residents, or a statement that their cost cannot be estimated; and

(4) a description of any matter in which the person:

(a) has been convicted of a felony, pleaded nolo contendere to a felony charge, or has been held liable or enjoined in a civil action by final judgment, if the felony or civil action involved fraud, embezzlement, fraudulent conversion, or misappropriation of property;

(b) is subject to an injunction or restrictive order of a court of record; or

(c) has had any state or federal license or permit suspended or revoked as a result of an action brought by a governmental agency if the order or action arose out of or was related to a business activity in a health care field, including an action affecting a license to operate a foster care facility, a nursing home, a retirement home, a home for the aged, or a facility subject to this chapter or a similar statute in another state.

Acts 1989, 71st Leg., ch. 678, Sec. 1, eff. Sept. 1, 1989.

Sec. 246.046. Contents of Disclosure Statement: Affiliation with Nonprofit Organization

The disclosure statement must state whether the provider is affiliated with a religious, charitable, or other nonprofit organization, and if so, the statement must:

(1) describe the extent of the affiliation;

(2) explain the extent to which the organization is responsible for the financial and contractual obligations of the provider; and

(3) cite any provision of the Internal Revenue Code of 1986 under which the provider or affiliate claims to be exempt from the payment of income tax.

Acts 1989, 71st Leg., ch. 678, Sec. 1, eff. Sept. 1, 1989.

Sec. 246.047. Contents of Disclosure Statement: Physical Property

(A) The disclosure statement must provide the location and a description of the proposed or existing physical property of the facility.

(B) If the physical property of the facility is proposed, the disclosure statement must state:

(1) the estimated completion date;
(2) whether construction has begun; and
(3) any contingencies under which construction may be deferred.

Acts 1989, 71st Leg., ch. 678, Sec. 1, eff. Sept. 1, 1989.

Sec. 246.048. Contents of Disclosure Statement: Contracts and Fees

The disclosure statement must describe:

(1) the services provided at the facility under a continuing care contract, including:
  (a) the extent to which medical care is furnished; and
  (b) those services that are included for specified basic fees for continuing care and those services that are made available at extra charge;
(2) all fees required of residents, including the entrance fee and any periodic charges;
(3) the conditions under which a continuing care contract at the facility may be canceled by the provider or the resident;
(4) any conditions under which all or part of the entrance fee is refundable on cancellation of the contract by the provider or the resident, or by the death of the resident before or during the occupancy of a living unit; and
(5) the manner by which the provider may adjust periodic charges or other recurring fees and any limitations on those adjustments.

Acts 1989, 71st Leg., ch. 678, Sec. 1, eff. Sept. 1, 1989.

Sec. 246.049. Contents of Disclosure Statement: Change of Circumstances

The disclosure statement must state:

(1) the policy of the facility regarding changes in the number of people residing in a living unit because of marriage or other relationships;

(2) the policy of the facility relating to the admission of a spouse to the facility and the consequences if the spouse does not meet the requirements for admission;

(3) the conditions under which a living unit occupied by a resident may be made available by the facility to a different resident other than on the death of the previous resident; and

(4) the health and financial conditions required for acceptance as a resident and for continuation as a resident, including the effect of any change in the health or financial condition of an individual between the date of the continuing care contract and the date on which the individual initially occupies a living unit.

Acts 1989, 71st Leg., ch. 678, Sec. 1, eff. Sept. 1, 1989.

Sec. 246.050. Contents of Disclosure Statement: Financial Information

(A) The disclosure statement must:

(1) describe any provisions made or to be made to provide reserve funding or security to enable the provider to fully perform its obligations under a continuing care contract at a facility, including:

  (a) the establishment of escrow accounts, trusts, or reserve funds and the manner in which those funds will be invested; and

(b) the name and experience of any individual in the direct employment of the provider who will make the investment decisions; and

(2) provide financial statements of the provider, including:

(a) a balance sheet as of the end of the most recent fiscal year; and

(b) income statements and a statement of cash flow for each of the three most recent fiscal years that the provider has been in existence.

(b) Financial statements required by Subsection (a)(2) must be prepared in accordance with generally accepted accounting principles and must be audited by an independent certified public accountant, who shall state in the audit report whether the financial statements were prepared in accordance with those principles.

Acts 1989, 71st Leg., ch. 678, Sec. 1, eff. Sept. 1, 1989. Amended by Acts 1991, 72nd Leg., ch. 14, Sec. 99, eff. Sept. 1, 1991.

Sec. 246.051. Contents of Disclosure Statement: Annual Income Statements

The disclosure statement must contain estimated annual income statements for the facility for at least five fiscal years, including:

(1) anticipated earning on any cash reserves;

(2) estimates of net receipts from entrance fees, other than entrance fees included in the statement of anticipated source and application of funds required under Section 246.052, minus estimated entrance fee refunds, including a description of the actuarial

basis and method of computation for the projection of entrance fee receipts;

(3) an estimate of gifts or bequests to be relied on to meet operating expenses;

(4) a projection of estimated income from fees and charges, excluding entrance fees, that:

(a) states individual rates anticipated to be charged; and

(b) includes a description of the assumptions used for computing the estimated occupancy rate of the facility and the effect on the income of the facility of any government subsidies for health care services to be provided under the continuing care contract;

(5) a projection of the facility's operating expenses, including:

(a) a description of the assumptions used in computing the expenses; and

(b) a separate allowance for the replacement of equipment and furnishings and anticipated major structural repairs or additions; and

(6) an estimate of annual payments of principal and interest required by a mortgage loan or other long-term financing arrangement relating to the facility.

Acts 1989, 71st Leg., ch. 678, Sec. 1, eff. Sept. 1, 1989. Amended by Acts 1991, 72nd Leg., ch. 14, Sec. 100, eff. Sept. 1, 1991.

Sec. 246.052. Contents of Disclosure Statement Anticipated Source and Application of Funds

If a facility has not begun operation, the disclosure statement must include a statement of the anticipated source and application of the funds to be used in the purchase or construction of the facility, including:

1. an estimate of the cost of purchasing or constructing and of equipping the facility, including financing expenses, legal expenses, land costs, occupancy development costs, and similar costs that the provider expects to incur or to become obligated to pay before operations begin;
2. a description of any mortgage loan or other long-term financing arrangement for the facility, including the anticipated terms and costs of the financing;
3. an estimate of the total entrance fees to be received from, or on behalf of, residents before the operation of the facility begins; and
4. an estimate of any funds anticipated to be necessary to cover initial losses and to provide reserve funds to assure full performance of the obligations of the provider under a continuing care contract.

Acts 1989, 71st Leg., ch. 678, Sec. 1, eff. Sept. 1, 1989.

Sec. 246.053. Standard Contract Form

(A) A copy of the standard contract form used by a provider must be attached as an exhibit to each disclosure statement.

(B) The standard contract form must specify the refund provisions of Sections 246.056 and 246.057.

Acts 1989, 71st Leg., ch. 678, Sec. 1, eff. Sept. 1, 1989. Amended by Acts 1991, 72nd Leg., ch. 14, Sec. 101, eff. Sept. 1, 1991.

Sec. 246.054. Annual Disclosure Statement Devision

(A) A provider shall file a revised disclosure statement

with the board not later than the 120th day after the date on which the provider's fiscal year ends.

(B) The revised disclosure statement must revise, as of the end of the provider's fiscal year, the information required by this subchapter.

(C) The revised disclosure statement must describe any material differences between:

(1) the estimated income statements filed under Section 246.052 as a part of the disclosure statement filed after the start of the provider's most recently completed fiscal year; and

(2) the actual result of operations during that fiscal year with the revised estimated income statements filed as a part of the revised disclosure statement.

(D) A provider may revise its disclosure statement and may file the revised disclosure statement at any other time if, in the provider's opinion, revision is necessary to prevent a disclosure statement from containing a material misstatement of fact or omitting a material fact required to be included in the disclosure statement.

(E) The commissioner shall review the disclosure statement for completeness but is not required to review the disclosure statement for accuracy.

Acts 1989, 71st Leg., ch. 678, Sec. 1, eff. Sept. 1, 1989.

Sec. 246.055. Advertisement in Conflict with Disclosures

A provider may not engage in any type of advertisement for a continuing care contract or facility if the advertisement contains a statement or representation in conflict with the disclosures required under this subchapter.

Acts 1989, 71st Leg., ch. 678, Sec. 1, eff. Sept. 1, 1989.

Sec. 246.056. Rescission of Contract; Required Language

(A) A person who executes a continuing care contract with a provider may rescind the contract at any time before the later of midnight of the seventh day, or a later day if specified in the contract:

(1) after the date on which the continuing care contract is executed; or

(2) after the date on which the person receives a disclosure statement that meets the requirements of this subchapter.

(B) A resident who executes a continuing care contract may not be required to move into the facility before the expiration of the period during which the contract may be rescinded.

(C) If a continuing care contract is rescinded under this section, any money or property transferred to the provider, other than periodic charges specified in the contract and applicable only to the period a living unit was actually occupied by the resident, shall be refunded not later than the 30th day after the date of rescission.

(D) Each continuing care contract must include the following statement or a substantially equivalent statement in type that is boldfaced, capitalized, underlined, or otherwise set out from the surrounding written material so as to be conspicuous:

> "You may cancel this contract at any time prior to midnight of the seventh day, or a later day if specified in the contract, after the date on which you sign this contract or you receive the facility's disclosure statement, whichever occurs later. If you elect to cancel the contract, you must do so by written notice and you will be entitled to receive a refund of all assets transferred other than periodic charges applicable to your occupancy of a living unit."

(E) Each continuing contract also must include the following statement in type that is boldfaced, capitalized, underlined, or otherwise set out from the surrounding written material so as to be conspicuous:

> "This document, if executed, constitutes a legal and binding contract between you and __________. You may wish to consult a legal or financial advisor before signing, although it is not required that you do so to make this contract binding."

Acts 1989, 71st Leg., ch. 678, Sec. 1, eff. Sept. 1, 1989. Amended by Acts 1991, 72nd Leg., ch. 14, Sec. 102, eff. Sept. 1, 1991; Acts 1993, 73rd Leg., ch. 953, Sec. 5, eff. Sept. 1, 1993.

Sec. 246.057. Cancellation of Contract: Death or Incapacity before Occupancy

(A) A continuing care contract is canceled if the resident:

(1) dies before occupying a living unit in the facility; or

(2) is precluded under the terms of the contract from occupying a living unit in the facility because of illness, injury, or incapacity.

(B) If a continuing care contract is canceled under this section, the resident or the resident's legal representative is entitled to a refund of all money or property transferred to the provider, minus:

(1) any nonstandard costs specifically incurred by the provider or facility at the request of the resident that are described in the contract or in an addendum to the contract signed by the resident; and

(2) a reasonable service charge, if set out in the contract, that may not exceed the greater of $1,000 or two percent of the entrance fee.

Acts 1989, 71st Leg., ch. 678, Sec. 1, eff. Sept. 1, 1989.

Amended by Acts 1993, 73rd Leg., ch. 953, Sec. 6, eff. Sept. 1, 1993.

Sec. 246.058. Disclosure Statement Fees

A facility that files a disclosure statement under Section 246.041 or 246.054 shall pay to the commissioner:

(1) a filing fee of $500; and

(2) a fee of not more than $2 for each living unit in the facility, excluding a unit devoted to that portion of the facility that is a licensed nursing home.

Acts 1989, 71st Leg., ch. 678, Sec. 1, eff. Sept. 1, 1989. Amended by Acts 1991, 72nd Leg., ch. 14, Sec. 103, eff. Sept. 1, 1991.

SUBCHAPTER D. ENTRANCE FEE AND RESERVE FUND ESCROW ACCOUNTS

Sec. 246.071. Entrance Fee Escrow Account; Escrow Agent

(A) Before a provider may accept the payment of a deposit made under a reservation agreement or any portion of an entrance fee, the provider must establish an entrance fee escrow account with a bank or trust company, as escrow agent, that is located in this state.

(B) The provider shall deposit with the escrow agent any deposit or any portion of an entrance fee received by the provider not later than 72 hours after the provider receives the deposit or fee.

Acts 1989, 71st Leg., ch. 678, Sec. 1, eff. Sept. 1, 1989. Amended by Acts 1993, 73rd Leg., ch. 953, Sec. 7, eff. Sept. 1, 1993.

Sec. 246.072. Return of Deposits; Release or Return of Entrance Fee

(A) On a written request from or on behalf of the provider or a prospective resident, the escrow agent shall return the amount on deposit to the person who paid the deposit or shall maintain the deposit as an entrance fee in the entrance fee escrow account.

(B) Unless the escrow agent receives a written request from or on behalf of a provider or a resident for the return of an entrance fee under Section 246.056, the agent shall release the fee to the provider or place the fee in a loan reserve fund escrow.

Acts 1989, 71st Leg., ch. 678, Sec. 1, eff. Sept. 1, 1989. Amended by Acts 1991, 72nd Leg., ch. 14, Sec. 104, eff. Sept. 1, 1991; Acts 1993, 73rd Leg., ch. 953, Sec. 8, eff. Sept. 1, 1993.

Sec. 246.073. Release to the Provider

(a) Except as provided by Subsection (b), an escrow agent shall release an entrance fee to the provider if:

(1) a minimum of 50 percent of the number of living units in the facility have been reserved for residents, as evidenced by:

- (a) uncanceled executed continuing care contracts with those residents; and
- (b) the receipt by the agent of entrance fee deposits of at least 10 percent of the entrance fee designated in each continuing care contract;

(2) the total amount of aggregate entrance fees received or receivable by the provider under binding continuing care contracts, the anticipated proceeds of any first mortgage loan or other long-term

financing commitment described under Subdivision (3), and funds from other sources in the actual possession of the provider are equal to or more than the total amount of:

(a) 90 percent of the aggregate cost of constructing or purchasing, equipping, and furnishing the facility;

(b) 90 percent of the funds estimated, in the statement of anticipated source and application of funds included in the disclosure statement, to be necessary to cover initial losses of the facility; and

(c) 90 percent of the amount of any loan reserve fund escrow required to be maintained by the provider under Section 246.077; and

(3) a commitment has been received by the provider for any permanent mortgage loan or other long-term financing described in the statement of anticipated source and application of funds included in the current disclosure statement and any conditions of the commitment before disbursement of funds have been substantially satisfied, other than completion of the construction or closing on the purchase of the facility; and:

(a) if construction of the facility has not been substantially completed:

(i) all necessary government permits or approvals have been obtained;

(ii) the provider and the general contractor responsible for construction of the facility have entered into a maximum price contract;

(iii) a recognized surety authorized to do business

in this state has executed in favor of the provider a bond covering faithful performance of the construction contract by the general contractor and the payment of all obligations under the contract;

(iv) the provider has entered a loan agreement for an interim construction loan in an amount that, when combined with the amount of entrance fees in escrow plus the amount of funds from other sources in the actual possession of the provider, equals or exceeds the estimated cost of constructing, equipping, and furnishing the facility;

(v) the lender has disbursed not less than 10 percent of the amount of the construction loan for physical construction or completed site preparation work; and

(vi) the provider has placed orders at firm prices for not less than 50 percent of the value of items necessary for equipping and furnishing the facility in accordance with the description in the disclosure statement, including any installation charges; or

(b) if construction or purchase of the facility has been substantially completed:

(i) an occupancy permit covering the living unit has been issued by the local government that has authority to issue the permit; and

(ii) if the entrance fee applies to a living unit that has been previously occupied, the living unit is available for occupancy by the new resident.

(b) Before the date on which the loan reserve fund escrow required under Section 246.077 is first established, the aggregate amount of entrance fees that may be released to the provider under this section may not exceed an amount equal to the aggregate amount of entrance fees received or receivable by the provider under binding continuing care contracts minus the amount of entrance fees received or receivable that are required to be maintained initially in the loan reserve fund escrow.

Acts 1989, 71st Leg., ch. 678, Sec. 1, eff. Sept. 1, 1989. Amended by Acts 1991, 72nd Leg., ch. 14, Sec. 105, eff. Sept. 1, 1991; Acts 1993, 73rd Leg., ch. 953, Sec. 9, eff. Sept. 1, 1993.

Sec. 246.074. Return of Entrance Fee

The escrow agent shall return an entrance fee to the person who paid it if the fee is not released to the provider or placed in the loan reserve fund escrow required under Section 246.077 within:

(1) 36 months after the date on which any portion of the entrance fee is received by the provider; or

(2) a longer time specified by the provider in the disclosure statement delivered with the continuing care contract under which the fee was paid.

Acts 1989, 71st Leg., ch. 678, Sec. 1, eff. Sept. 1, 1989. Amended by Acts 1991, 72nd Leg., ch. 14, Sec. 106, eff. Sept. 1, 1991; Acts 1993, 73rd Leg., ch. 953, Sec. 10, eff. Sept. 1, 1993.

Sec. 246.075. Escrow of Application Fee not Required

This subchapter does not require the escrow of any nonrefundable portion of a deposit or entrance fee that:

(1) does not exceed an amount equal to two percent of the entrance fee; and

(2) is clearly designated as nonrefundable in the continuing care contract or reservation agreement.

Acts 1989, 71st Leg., ch. 678, Sec. 1, eff. Sept. 1, 1989. Amended by Acts 1993, 73rd Leg., ch. 953, Sec. 11, eff. Sept. 1, 1993.

Sec. 246.076. Interest Accrued on Entrance Fee Funds

Unless otherwise provided in a continuing care contract, interest that accrues on funds held in an entrance fee escrow account is the property of the provider.

Acts 1989, 71st Leg., ch. 678, Sec. 1, eff. Sept. 1, 1989. Amended by Acts 1993, 73rd Leg., ch. 953, Sec. 12, eff. Sept. 1, 1993.

Sec. 246.077. Reserve Fund Escrow

(A) When a facility is first occupied by a resident, the provider shall establish and maintain in an escrow account with a bank or trust company, as escrow agent, that is located in this state a reserve fund equal to the total of all principal and interest payments due during the next 12 months on any first mortgage loan or other long-term financing arrangement for the facility. The requirements of this section may be met in whole or in part by other reserve funds held for the purpose of meeting loan obligations if the total amount equals or exceeds the amount required by this subsection.

(B) At the option of the facility, the loan reserve fund escrow amount may exclude the portion of principal and interest payments applicable to that portion of the facility that is a licensed nursing home.

(C) The provider shall maintain the loan reserve fund

escrow in an account that is fully covered by federal deposit insurance and is separate from the provider's business account or in other accounts or investments approved by the commissioner. The funds in the reserve fund escrow account may be invested, with earnings payable to the provider.

Acts 1989, 71st Leg., ch. 678, Sec. 1, eff. Sept. 1, 1989. Amended by Acts 1991, 72nd Leg., ch. 14, Sec. 107, eff. Sept. 1, 1991.

Sec. 246.078. Release of Reserve Fund Escrow

(A) The escrow agent may release an amount equal to not more than one-twelfth of the loan reserve fund required by Section 246.077 if the provider requests the release in writing.

(B) The escrow agent must give written notice to the board not later than the 11th day before the date of the release.

(C) The escrow agent may not release funds from the loan reserve fund escrow under this section more than once during a calendar year. A provider at any time may apply to the commissioner for the withdrawal of all or part of the loan reserve escrow funds. The provider may withdraw the funds on the approval of the withdrawal by the commissioner. The application must be made and the approval given as provided by rule.

(D) The provider must repay to the loan reserve fund escrow account the amount released to the provider under Subsection (a) or (c) not later than 18 months after the date the amount is released. The commissioner may place the provider or facility under supervision under Section 246.091 or take any other appropriate action as provided by law if the provider does not repay the loan reserve fund escrow account within the required period.

Acts 1989, 71st Leg., ch. 678, Sec. 1, eff. Sept. 1, 1989. Amended by Acts 1991, 72nd Leg., ch. 14, Sec. 108, eff. Sept. 1, 1991.

Sec. 246.079. Transition

(A) A provider who operates a facility that existed on September 1, 1987, must comply with the filing requirements imposed under Section 246.041 and the escrow requirements imposed under Sections 246.077 and 246.078 not later than September 1, 1990.

(B) The commissioner may extend the time for compliance under this section for a reasonable period if the commissioner determines that the provider is unable to comply with this section after making a good faith effort to comply.

Acts 1989, 71st Leg., ch. 678, Sec. 1, eff. Sept. 1, 1989. Amended by Acts 1991, 72nd Leg., ch. 14, Sec. 109, eff. Sept. 1, 1991.

Sec. 246.080. Applicability

Sections 246.071 through 246.076 do not apply to a facility that on September 1, 1987, was completed and occupied by at least one person.

Added by Acts 1991, 72nd Leg., ch. 14, Sec. 110, eff. Sept. 1, 1991.

SUBCHAPTER E. SUPERVISION, REHABILITATION, AND LIQUIDATION

Sec. 246.091. Supervision by Commissioner

(A) The commissioner may place a provider or facility under supervision if:

(1) the provider draws on the provider's entrance fee escrow in an amount greater than permitted by Section 246.073;

(2) the provider draws on the provider's loan reserve fund escrow in an amount greater than permitted or more frequently than permitted by Section 246.078;

(3) the commissioner determines, after a complaint and investigation, that the provider is financially unsound or is unable to meet the income or available cash projections previously filed by the provider and that the ability of the provider to fully perform its obligations under continuing care contracts is endangered; or

(4) the provider is bankrupt, insolvent, or has filed for protection from creditors under a federal or state reorganization, bankruptcy, or insolvency law.

(B) The commissioner appoints the supervisor.

(C) The commissioner may provide that the provider may not, during the supervision period and without the prior approval of the commissioner or the supervisor:

(1) dispose of, convey, or encumber its assets;

(2) withdraw its bank accounts;

(3) lend its funds;

(4) invest its funds;

(5) transfer its property;

(6) incur a debt, obligation, or liability; or

(7) merge or consolidate with another facility.

(D) The commissioner shall terminate the supervision and restore to a provider the authority to manage the affairs of the facility if the commissioner determines that the facility is capable of meeting its financial obligations.

(E) The facility or provider shall pay the costs of a supervisor.

Acts 1989, 71st Leg., ch. 678, Sec. 1, eff. Sept. 1, 1989. Amended by Acts 1991, 72nd Leg., ch. 14, Sec. 111, eff. Sept. 1, 1991.

Sec. 246.092. Application for Court Order for Rehabilitation or Liquidation

(A) The commissioner shall request the attorney general to apply to a district court of this state, or to the federal bankruptcy court that has exercised jurisdiction over a provider or facility, for an order directing the appointment of a trustee to rehabilitate or liquidate the facility if the commissioner elects not to place the facility under supervision and:

(1) the provider draws from the provider's loan reserve fund escrow an amount greater than permitted by Section 246.078;

(2) the provider does not repay the loan reserve fund escrow as required by Section 246.078;

(3) the board determines, after a complaint and investigation, that the provider is financially unsound or is unable to meet the income or available cash projections previously filed by the provider and that the ability of the provider to fully perform its obligations under continuing care contracts is endangered; or

(4) the provider is bankrupt, insolvent, or has filed for protection from creditors under a federal or state reorganization, bankruptcy, or insolvency law.

(B) In connection with an application for an order to rehabilitate or liquidate a facility, the court shall consider the manner in which the welfare of persons who have previously contracted with the provider for continuing care at the facility may be best served, and may order that the proceeds of a lien imposed under Section 246.111 may be used in full or partial payment of entrance fees to other facilities on behalf of the residents of the facility being liquidated.

Acts 1989, 71st Leg., ch. 678, Sec. 1, eff. Sept. 1, 1989. Amended by Acts 1991, 72nd Leg., ch. 14, Sec. 112, eff. Sept. 1, 1991.

Sec. 246.093. Order to Rehabilitate

An order to rehabilitate a facility must direct the trustee to:

(1) take possession of the provider's property in order to conduct the business, including employing any managers or agents the trustee considers necessary; and

(2) take action as directed by the court to eliminate the causes and conditions that made rehabilitation necessary.

Acts 1989, 71st Leg., ch. 678, Sec. 1, eff. Sept. 1, 1989.

Sec. 246.094. Order to Liquidate

(A) If the trustee determines that further efforts to rehabilitate the provider would be impractical or useless, the trustee may apply to the court that ordered the rehabilitation for an order of liquidation.

(B) A court that has jurisdiction may issue an order to liquidate a facility on application of the board, regardless of whether an order to rehabilitate the facility exists. If the court issues an order to liquidate, the court shall appoint a trustee to collect and liquidate all of the provider's assets located in this state.

(C) A person may not contract for continuing care at a

facility after an order to liquidate that facility has been entered.

Acts 1989, 71st Leg., ch. 678, Sec. 1, eff. Sept. 1, 1989.

Sec. 246.095. Bond

A court may refuse to make or may vacate an order to rehabilitate under this subchapter if the provider posts a bond that is:

(1) in an amount determined by the court to be equal to the reserve funding needed to fulfill the provider's obligations under its continuing care contracts at the facility;

(2) issued by a recognized surety authorized to do business in this state; and

(3) executed in favor of the state on behalf of all persons entitled to refunds of entrance fees from the provider or other damages if the provider is unable to fulfill its continuing care contracts at the facility.

Acts 1989, 71st Leg., ch. 678, Sec. 1, eff. Sept. 1, 1989.

Sec. 246.096. Termination of Rehabilitation

(A) A court may terminate a rehabilitation and order return of a facility and its assets and affairs to the management of the provider if the court, on petition of the trustee or the provider or on its own motion, finds that:

(1) the objectives of the order to rehabilitate the facility have been accomplished; and

(2) the facility can be returned to the provider's management without further jeopardy to the residents, creditors, or owners of the facility or the public.

(B) A court may enter an order under this section after:

(1) a full report and accounting of the conduct of the facility's affairs during the rehabilitation; and

(2) a report on the facility's financial condition.

Acts 1989, 71st Leg., ch. 678, Sec. 1, eff. Sept. 1, 1989.

Sec. 246.097. Payment of Trustee

The reasonable costs, expenses, and fees of the trustee are payable from the assets of the facility.

Acts 1989, 71st Leg., ch. 678, Sec. 1, eff. Sept. 1, 1989.

SUBCHAPTER F. ENFORCEMENT

Sec. 246.111. Lien

(a) To secure the obligations of the provider under any continuing care contract, a lien attaches on the date a resident first occupies a facility. The lien covers the real and personal property of the provider located at the facility. The provider shall prepare a written notice sworn to by an officer of the provider for each county where the provider has a facility. The notice must contain the name of the provider, the legal description of each facility of the provider, and a statement that the facility is subject to this chapter and the lien provided by this section. The provider shall file for record the notice in the real property records of each county where the provider has a facility on or before the later of January 1, 1994, or the date of the execution of the first continuing care contract relating to the facility.

(b) The commissioner may remove a lien under this section if requested by a provider to obtain secondary financing or refinancing of a facility if:

(1) the facility is financially sound; and

(2) removal of the lien does not adversely affect the residents.

(c) A lien under this section is subordinate to any liens on the property of the facility if the proceeds of the loan secured by the liens were used in whole or in part to:

(1) construct, acquire, replace, or improve the facility; or

(2) refinance an earlier loan used to construct, acquire, replace, or improve the facility.

(d) A lien under this section is effective for 10 years.

(e) A lien under this section may be foreclosed on application of the board if the facility is liquidated or the provider is insolvent or bankrupt. The proceeds from a foreclosed lien shall be used for full or partial satisfaction of the provider's obligations under continuing care contracts in effect on the date of the foreclosure.

Acts 1989, 71st Leg., ch. 678, Sec. 1, eff. Sept. 1, 1989. Amended by Acts 1993, 73rd Leg., ch. 953, Sec. 13, 15, eff. Sept. 1, 1993.

Sec. 246.112. Investigations

The commissioner may conduct an examination or investigation as necessary to:

(1) determine whether a person has violated or is about to violate this chapter;

(2) aid in the enforcement of this chapter;

(3) determine the financial solvency of a facility; or

(4) verify a statement contained in a disclosure statement filed or delivered under this chapter.

Acts 1989, 71st Leg., ch. 678, Sec. 1, eff. Sept. 1, 1989.

Sec. 246.113. Production of Evidence

(A) In an investigation or proceeding under this chapter, the board may:

(1) require or allow a person to file a written statement regarding any of the facts and circumstances concerning the matter to be investigated;

(2) administer oaths and affirmations;

(3) subpoena witnesses;

(4) compel attendance;

(5) take evidence; and

(6) require the production of any books, papers, correspondence, memoranda, agreements, or other documents or records considered relevant to the inquiry.

(B) The board may bring suit in district court to enforce a subpoena if the person to whom a subpoena is directed fails to comply.

Acts 1989, 71st Leg., ch. 678, Sec. 1, eff. Sept. 1, 1989.

Sec. 246.114. Actuarial Review

(A) This section applies only to a facility whose contracts offer future guarantees of long-term nursing care that develop current actuarial liabilities.

(B) A facility subject to this section that initially filed with the commissioner an actuarial review performed on or after September 1, 1982, and before September 1, 1987, shall file with the commissioner subsequent actuarial reviews at five-year intervals from the date of completion of the initial actuarial review.

(C) A facility subject to this section that initially filed with the commissioner an actuarial review performed on or after September 1, 1987, shall file with the commissioner subsequent actuarial reviews at five-year intervals from the date of the filing of the initial actuarial review.

(D) The commissioner may require an actuarial review of a facility before the end of the five-year interval in which the facility would otherwise be required to file an actuarial review if, in the opinion of the commissioner, the facility exhibits conditions of financial instability warranting an earlier review.

Acts 1989, 71st Leg., ch. 678, Sec. 1, eff. Sept. 1, 1989. Amended by Acts 1991, 72nd Leg., ch. 14, Sec. 113, eff. Sept. 1, 1991; Acts 1993, 73rd Leg., ch. 953, Sec. 14, eff. Sept. 1, 1993.

Sec. 246.115. Cease and Desist Orders; in Junctions

(A) The board may request that the attorney general bring an action to prohibit a person from engaging in an act or practice and to order compliance with this chapter if the board determines, after a complaint or by other means, that the act or practice violates this chapter or an order made under this chapter.

(B) The action may be brought in the district court of a county in which:

(1) the defendant resides;
(2) the defendant has done business;
(3) the principal place of business of the defendant is located; or
(4) the transaction occurred.

(C) The court may grant an injunction or restraining order on a proper showing. If the court grants an injunction or restraining order, the court shall issue it without bond.

Acts 1989, 71st Leg., ch. 678, Sec. 1, eff. Sept. 1, 1989.

Sec. 246.116. Criminal Penalty

(A) A person commits an offense if the person intentionally violates this chapter.

(B) An offense under this section is a Class A misdemeanor.

Acts 1989, 71st Leg., ch. 678, Sec. 1, eff. Sept. 1, 1989.

Sec. 246.117. Civil Liability

(A) A provider who makes a continuing care contract without complying with the disclosure statement requirement under Subchapter C, or who makes a continuing care contract with a person who has relied on a disclosure statement that omits a material fact required to be stated in the statement or necessary to make the statement accurate, is liable to the person with whom the continuing care contract is made for:

(1) actual damages;

(2) repayment of all fees paid to the provider minus the reasonable value of care and lodging provided to the person by or on whose behalf the continuing care contract was made before the violation, misstatement, or omission was discovered or reasonably should have been discovered;

(3) interest at the legal rate for judgments;

(4) court costs; and

(5) reasonable attorney's fees.

(B) A provider is liable under this section regardless of whether the provider had actual knowledge of the misstatement or omission.

(C) A person may not file or maintain an action under this section if the person, before filing the action, received a written offer of a refund of all amounts paid to the provider, facility, or person violating this chapter and reasonable interest from the date of payment, minus the reasonable value of care and lodging provided before the receipt of the offer and:

(1) the offer states the provisions of this section; and

(2) the recipient of the offer fails to accept the offer within 30 days after the date the offer is received.

(D) A person must bring suit under this section not later than three years after:

(1) the date on which the continuing care contract was entered into; or

(2) the violation, misstatement, or omission is discovered or reasonably should have been discovered.

(D) Except as expressly provided by this chapter, civil liability does not arise in favor of a private party by implication from or as a result of the violation of this chapter or a rule or order adopted under this chapter.

(F) This chapter does not limit a liability that would exist under any other statute or common law if this chapter were not in effect.

(G) The provisions of this chapter are not exclusive and the remedies provided by this chapter are in addition to any other remedies provided by any other law.

Acts 1989, 71st Leg., ch. 678, Sec. 1, eff. Sept. 1, 1989.

CHAPTER 284. SPECIAL PROVISIONS RELATING TO HOSPITAL DISTRICT BONDS

SUBCHAPTER A. ISSUANCE OF REVENUE BONDS IN COUNTIES WITH POPULATION OF AT LEAST 200,000

Sec. 284.001. Authority to Issue; Frm of Bonds

(a) The commissioners court of a county with a population of at least 200,000 in which a hospital district has been created in accordance with Article IX of the Texas Constitution may issue revenue bonds to provide funds to:

(1) acquire, construct, repair, renovate, improve, enlarge, and equip a hospital facility; and

(2) acquire any real or personal property on behalf of the district for those purposes.

(b) The commissioners court may not issue revenue bonds under this subchapter on behalf of a hospital district to purchase a nursing home for long-term care.

(c) The bonds and bond interest coupons are negotiable instruments.

(d) The bonds may be issued in the form, denomination, and manner and under the terms and conditions determined and provided by the commissioners court in the order authorizing the issuance of the bonds.

Acts 1989, 71st Leg., ch. 678, Sec. 1, eff. Sept. 1, 1989.

Sec. 284.002. Terms

(a) The bonds must mature serially or otherwise not more than 40 years after the date they are issued.

(b) The bonds may be:

(1) made redeemable before maturity; and

(2) issued registrable as to principal or as to principal and interest.

(c) The bonds shall be executed in the manner and bear interest at the rate provided by the commissioners court in the order authorizing the bonds.

Acts 1989, 71st Leg., ch. 678, Sec. 1, eff. Sept. 1, 1989.

Sec. 284.003. Approval and Registration of Bonds

(a) The commissioners court shall submit the bonds and the proceedings authorizing their issuance to the attorney general for examination. If the attorney general finds that the bonds are authorized in accordance with law, the attorney general shall approve the bonds and the comptroller shall register the bonds.

(b) After approval and registration, the bonds are incontestable and are binding obligations according to their terms.

Acts 1989, 71st Leg., ch. 678, Sec. 1, eff. Sept. 1, 1989.

Sec. 284.004. Security

(a) The commissioners court may make bonds issued under this subchapter payable from and secured by a lien on or pledge of all or part of the hospital district revenue from operation or ownership of hospital facilities, except ad valorem taxes.

(b) The commissioners court may also secure the bonds by:

(1) a pledge of all or part of a grant, a donation, or other income received from a public or private source, whether in accordance with an agreement or otherwise; and

(2) a mortgage or deed of trust on real property on

which a district hospital facility is or will be located and any real or personal property incident or appurtenant to that facility.

(c) The commissioners court may authorize the execution and delivery of a trust indenture, mortgage, deed of trust, or other form of encumbrance to evidence a security agreement under Subsection (b)(2).

Acts 1989, 71st Leg., ch. 678, Sec. 1, eff. Sept. 1, 1989.

Sec. 284.005. Sale of Bonds; Use of Proceeds

(a) The bonds may be sold in the manner, at the price, and under the terms determined and provided by the commissioners court in the order authorizing the issuance of the bonds.

(b) If permitted by the bond order, a required part of the proceeds from the bond sale may be used for:

(1) the payment of interest on the bonds during the construction of hospital facilities financed with bond proceeds;

(2) the payment of operation and maintenance expenses of those facilities to the extent and for the period specified by the bond order; and

(3) the creation of reserves for the payment of bond principal and interest.

Acts 1989, 71st Leg., ch. 678, Sec. 1, eff. Sept. 1, 1989.

Sec. 284.006. Investment of Bond Proceeds

Proceeds from the sale of bonds may be invested until needed to the extent and in the manner provided by the bond order.

Acts 1989, 71st Leg., ch. 678, Sec. 1, eff. Sept. 1, 1989.

Sec. 284.007. Legal Investments

The bonds are legal and authorized investments for:

(1) a bank;

(2) a trust company;

(3) a savings and loan association;

(4) an insurance company;

(5) a small business investment corporation;

(6) a fiduciary;

(7) a trustee;

(8) a guardian; or

(9) an interest or sinking fund or other public funds of the state or a municipality, county, school district, or other political subdivision of the state.

Acts 1989, 71st Leg., ch. 678, Sec. 1, eff. Sept. 1, 1989.

Sec. 284.008. Security for Deposits

The bonds are eligible to secure deposits of public funds of the state or of a municipality, county, school district, or other political subdivision of the state. The bonds are lawful and sufficient security for deposits to the extent of their market value if accompanied by all appurtenant unmatured coupons, if any.

Acts 1989, 71st Leg., ch. 678, Sec. 1, eff. Sept. 1, 1989.

Sec. 284.009. Authority to Issue Subsequent Bonds

In the authorization of bonds under Section 284.001, the commissioners court may provide for the subsequent issuance of additional parity, subordinate lien, or other bonds, under the terms or conditions stated in the order authorizing the issuance of the original bonds.

Acts 1989, 71st Leg., ch. 678, Sec. 1, eff. Sept. 1, 1989.

Sec. 284.010. Refunding Bonds and Refinancing

(a) Revenue bonds issued by the commissioners court under this subchapter or under any other statute of this state and payable from hospital facility revenue may be refunded or otherwise refinanced by the commissioners court.

(b) The provisions of this subchapter pertinent and appropriate to the issuance of revenue bonds generally apply to the refunding bonds.

(c) In issuing refunding bonds or in refinancing revenue bonds, the commissioners court in the same authorizing proceedings may:

(1) refund or refinance bonds issued under this subchapter and bonds issued under another statute of this state and combine the refunding bonds with other new bonds to be issued under those laws into one or more issues or series of bonds; and

(2) provide for the subsequent issuance of additional parity, subordinate lien, or other bonds.

(d) Refunding bonds shall be issued and delivered under the terms and conditions stated in the authorizing proceedings.

Acts 1989, 71st Leg., ch. 678, Sec. 1, eff. Sept. 1, 1989.

Sec. 284.011. Taxes to Pay Operating and Maintenance Expenses

(a) Ad valorem taxes of the hospital district shall be used to pay hospital facility operation and maintenance expenses to the extent that hospital facility revenue and income are not available at any time to pay all those expenses.

(b) The proceeds of an annual ad valorem tax may be pledged to pay hospital facility operation and maintenance expenses in the order authorizing the issuance of bonds under this subchapter.

(c) During each year that any of the bonds are outstanding, the commissioners court shall compute and determine the rate and amount of ad valorem tax that is sufficient to raise and produce the funds required to pay required hospital facility operation and maintenance expenses if the annual ad valorem tax is pledged as security for the payment of those expenses. In determining the tax rate, the commissioners court may allow for tax delinquencies and the cost of tax collection.

Acts 1989, 71st Leg., ch. 678, Sec. 1, eff. Sept. 1, 1989.

Sec. 284.012. Authority of District Governing Body in Absence of Ad Val Orem Tax

If a hospital district created under Article IX of the Texas Constitution does not have ad valorem taxes levied on behalf of the district by the commissioners court of the county in which the hospital district is located, the district board of directors or other governing body has all of the powers and duties otherwise provided to a commissioners court under this subchapter.

Acts 1989, 71st Leg., ch. 678, Sec. 1, eff. Sept. 1, 1989.

Sec. 284.013. Annual Budget

(a) The commissioners court, board of hospital managers, or hospital district board of directors shall provide in each annual hospital district budget for the payment of all operation and maintenance expenses of the hospital district.

(b) In preparing the budget, the commissioners court or board may consider the estimated revenue and income from hospital facilities that will be available for paying operation and maintenance expenses after providing for all principal, interest, and reserve requirements in connection with the bonds.

Acts 1989, 71st Leg., ch. 678, Sec. 1, eff. Sept. 1, 1989.

Sec. 284.014. Authority to Charge for Hospital Services

(a) The commissioners court, board of hospital managers, or hospital district board of directors may fix and collect charges for the occupancy or use of hospital facilities and hospital services in the amount and manner determined by the commissioners court or board.

(b) The charges shall be fixed and collected in an amount:

(1) sufficient, with other pledged resources, to provide for all payments of principal, interest, and any other amounts required in connection with the bonds; and

(2) required by the bond order to provide for payment of all or part of the operation, maintenance, and other expenses of the hospital facilities.

Acts 1989, 71st Leg., ch. 678, Sec. 1, eff. Sept. 1, 1989.

Sec. 284.015. Use of SE OF Other Law

A commissioners court may use other law not in conflict with this chapter to the extent convenient or necessary to carry out any power expressly or impliedly granted by this chapter.

Acts 1989, 71st Leg., ch. 678, Sec. 1, eff. Sept. 1, 1989.

SUBCHAPTER B. ISSUING AND REFUNDING REVENUE BONDS BY HOSPITAL DISTRICTS CREATED UNDER ARTICLE IX, SECTION 9, OF THE TEXAS CONSTITUTION

Sec. 284.031. Authority to Issue

(a) A hospital district created in accordance with Article IX, Section 9, of the Texas Constitution may issue revenue bonds to:

(1) acquire, construct, repair, renovate, or equip buildings and improvements for hospital purposes; and

(2) acquire sites for hospital purposes.

(b) The hospital district may refund revenue bonds previously issued for the purposes specified by Subsection (a).

(c) The bonds must be payable from and secured by a pledge of all or part of district revenues from operation of a hospital. The bonds may also be secured by a mortgage or deed of trust lien on all or part of the district's property.

(d) The bonds must be issued in accordance with Sections 264.042-264.047(a), 264.048, and 264.049, and with the effect specified by Section 264.050.

Acts 1989, 71st Leg., ch. 678, Sec. 1, eff. Sept. 1, 1989.

SUBCHAPTER C. BOND ELECTIONS IN HOSPITAL DISTRICTS

Sec. 284.041. Bond Elections for Revenue Bonds

(a) The commissioners court of a county authorized by law to issue revenue bonds on behalf of a hospital district in the county may, on its own motion, order an advisory election to determine whether a majority of the qualified voters of the hospital district voting at the election favor the issuance of revenue bonds. The order must contain the same information contained in the notice of the election.

(b) In addition to the contents of the notice required by the Election Code, the notice must state any other matters that the commissioners court considers necessary or advisable.

(c) Subject to any additional notice requirements under Section 4.003, Election Code, the commissioners court shall publish notice of the election one time, at least 10 days before the date set for the election, in a newspaper of general circulation in the hospital district.

(d) The election is advisory only and does not affect the authority of the commissioners court to issue revenue bonds on behalf of the hospital district under an applicable law that does not require an election.

(e) The expenses of holding the election shall be paid from hospital district funds.

Acts 1989, 71st Leg., ch. 678, Sec. 1, eff. Sept. 1, 1989.

Bibliography

American Hospital Association (AHA). 1966. *Housekeeping Manual for Health Care Facilities.* AHA: Chicago.

American Medical Association Council on Scientific Affairs. 1985. "Guidelines for handling parenteral antineoplastics." *J.A.M.A.* 253:1590-2.

American National Standards Institute (ANSI). 1982. *Standard for Anesthetic Equipment-Scavenging Systems for Excess Anesthetic Gases.* ANSI Z79.11-1982.

American National Standards Institute (ANSI). 1988. *Standard for the Safe Use of Lasers in Health Care Facilities.* ANSI Z136.3-1988.

American National Standards Institute. 1968. *Occupational and Educational Eye and Face Protection.* ANSI Z87.1.

American Society of Hospital Pharmacists. 1990. ASHP Technical Assistance Bulletin on Handling Cytotoxic and Hazardous Drugs. *Am. J. Hosp. Pharm.* 47:1033-49.

Andersen, R., Boedicker, M., Ma, M., and Goldstein, E.J.C. 1986. "Adverse Reactions Associated with Pentamidine Isethionate in AIDS Patients: Recommendations for Monitoring Therapy." *Drug Intell. Clin. Pharm.* 20:862-8.

Anderson, R.W., Puckett, W.H., Dana, W.J., et al. 1982. "Risk of handling injectable antineoplastic agents." *Am. J. Hosp. Pharm.* 39:1881-87.

Avis, K.E., and Levchuck, J.W. 1984. "Special considerations in the use of vertical laminar flow workbenches." *Am. J. Hosp. Pharm.* 41:81-7.

Barber, R.K. 1981. "Fetal and neonatal effects of cytotoxic agents." *Obstet. Gynecol.* 51:41S-47S.

Benhamou, S., Pot-Deprun, J., Sancho-Garnier, H., and Chouroulinkov, I. 1988. "Sister chromatid exchanges and chromosomal aberrations in lymphocytes of nurses handling cytostatic drugs." I 41:350-3.

Bos, R.P., Leenars, A.O., Theuws, J.L., and Henderson, P.T. 1982. "Mutagenicity of urine from nurses handling cytostatic drugs, influence of smoking." *Int. Arch. Occ. Envir.* Health 50:359-69.

Bryan, D., and Marback, R.C. 1984. "Laminar-airflow equipment certification: What the pharmacist needs to know." *Am. J. Hosp. Pharm.* 41:1343-9.

Burgaz, S., Ozdamar, Y.N., and Karakaya, A.E. 1988. "A signal assay for the detection of genotoxic compounds: Application on the urine of cancer patients on chemotherapy and of nurses handling cytotoxic drugs." *Human Toxicol.* 7:557-60.

California Department of Health Services Occupational Health Surveillance and Evaluation Program. 1986. "Health care worker exposure to ribavirin aerosol: field investigation Fl-86-009." Berkeley: California Department of Health Services.

Castegnaro, M., Adams, J., Armour, M.A., et al., eds. 1985. *Laboratory decontamination and destruction of carcinogens in laboratory wastes: Some antineoplastic agents.* International Agency for Research on Cancer. Scientific Publications No. 73. Lyon, France: IARC.

Chaff, L.F. 1989. *Safety Guide for Healthcare Institutions.* 4th ed. American Hospital Publishing: Chicago.

Chapman, R.M. 1984. "Effect of cytotoxic therapy on sexuality and gonadal function." In *Toxicity of Chemotherapy.* Perry, M.C. and J.W. Yarbro (eds.). 343-363. Orlando: Grune & Stratton.

Charney, W. and Schirmer, J. 1990. *Essentials of Modern Hospital Safety.* Lewis Publishers, Inc.: Chelsea, MI.

Chen, C.H., Vazquez-Padua, M., and Cheng, Y.C. 1990. "Effect of anti-human immunodeficiency virus nucleoside analogs on mDNA and its implications for delayed toxicity." *Mol. Pharm.* 39:625-628.

Christensen, C.J., Lemasters, G.K., and Wakeman, M.A. 1990. "Work practices and policies of hospital pharmacists preparing antineoplastic agents." *J. Occup. Med.* 32:508-12.

Chrysostomou, A., Morley, A.A., and Seshadri, R. 1984. "Mutation frequency in nurses and pharmacists working with cytotoxic drugs." *Aust. N.Z.J. Med.* 14:831-4.

Connor, J.D., Hintz, M., and Van Dyke, R. 1984. "Ribavirin pharmacokinetics in children and adults during therapeutic trials." In Clinical Applications of Ribavirin, Smith, R.A., Knight, V., and Smith, J.A.D. (eds.) Orlando: Academic Press.

Connor, T.H., Laidlaw, J.L., Theiss, J.C., et al. 1984. "Permeability of latex and polyvinyl chloride gloves to carmustine." *Am. J. Hosp. Pharm.* 41:676-9.

Crudi, C.B. 1980. "A compounding dilemma: I've kept the drug sterile but have I contaminated myself?" *Nat. Intra. Therapy J.* 3:77-80.

Department of Health and Human Services. *Healthy people 2000: national health promotion and disease prevention objectives.* Washington, DC: U. S. Department of Health and Human Services;. 1990. (Full Text in PMC)

Doll, D.C. 1989. Aerosolised pentamidine. Lancet ii:1284-5.

Duvall, E., and Baumann, B. 1980. "An unusual accident during the administration of chemotherapy." *Cancer Nurs.* 3:305-6.

ECRI. 1989. *Ethylene Oxide: Protecting Your Employees.* Hospital Hazardous Management. Vol. 1, Nos. 1 & 2, Contact ECRI at 5200 Butler Pike, Plymouth Meeting, PA 19462, (215) 825-6000.

ECRI. 1989. *Ethylene Oxide: Protecting Your Employees.* Hospital Hazardous Management. Vol. 1, Nos. 1 & 2, Contact ECRI at 5200 Butler Pike, Plymouth Meeting, PA 19462, (215) 825-6000.

Environmental Protection Agency. 1991. *Discarded commercial chemical products, off specification species, container residues, and spill residues thereof.* 40 CFR 261.33(f).

Everson, R.B., Ratcliffe, J.M., Flack, P.M., et al. 1985. "Detection of low levels of urinary mutagen excretion by chemotherapy workers which was not related to occupational drug exposures." *Cancer Research* 45:6487-97.

Falck, K., Grohn, P., Sorsa, M., et al. 1979. "Mutagenicity in urine of nurses handling cytostatic drugs." *Lancet* i:1250-1.

Falck, K., Sorsa, M., and Vainio, H. 1981. "Use of the bacterial fluctation test to detect mutagenicity in urine of nurses handling cytostatic drugs." (abstract). *Mutation Res.* 85:236-7.

Ferguson, L.R., Everts, R., Robbie, M.A., et al. 1988. "The use within New Zealand of cytogenetic approaches to monitoring of hospital pharmacists for exposure to cytotoxic drugs: Report of a pilot study in Auckland." *Aust J Hosp Pharm.* 18:228-33.

Gude, J.K. 1989. "Selective delivery of pentamidine to the lung by aerosol." *Am. Rev. Resp. Dis.* 139:1060.

Guglielmo, B.J., Jacobs, R.A., and Locksley, R.M. 1989. "The exposure of health care workers to ribavirin aerosol." *J.A.M.A.* 261:1880-1.

Harrison, R., Bellows, J., Rempel, D., et al. 1988. "Assessing exposures of health-care personnel to aerosols of ribavirin — California." *Morbidity and Mortality Weekly Report* 37:560-3.

Hemminki, K., Kyyronen, P., and Lindbohm, M.L. 1985. "Spontaneous abortions and malformations in the offspring of nurses exposed to anaesthetic gases, cytostatic drugs, and other potential hazards in hospitals, based on registered information of outcome." *J. Epidem. Comm.* Health 39:141-7.

Henderson, D.K., and Gerberding, J.L. 1989. "Prophylactic zidovudine after occupational exposure to the human immunodeficiency virus: An interim analysis." *J. Infectious Diseases* 160:321-7.

Hillyard, I. W. 1980. "The preclinical toxicology and safety of ribavirin." In Ribavirin: a broad spectrum antiviral agent. Smith, R.A., and Kirkpatrick, W. (eds.) New York: Academic Press.

Hirst, M., Tse, S., Mills, D.G., et al. 1984. "Occupational exposure to cyclophosphamide." *Lancet* 1:186-8.

Hoeltge, G.A. 1986. *Documentation of Safe Work Practices in the Clinical Laboratory*. Clinics in Laboratory Medicine 6(4):787-798.

Hoy, R.H. and Stump, L.M. 1984. "Effect of an air-venting filter device on aerosol production from vials." *Am. J. Hosp. Pharm.* 41:324-6.

International Agency for Research on Cancer. 1981. *IARC*

Monographs on the Evaluation of the Carcinogenic Risk of Chemicals to Humans: Some Antineoplastic and Immunosuppressive Agents. Vol. 26. Lyon, France: IARC.

International Agency for Research on Cancer. 1987. *IARC Monographs on the Evaluation of the Carcinogenic Risk of Chemicals to Humans; Genetic and related effects: An updating of selected IARC Monographs from Volumes 1-42.* Vol. 1-42 (Suppl. 6). Lyon, France: IARC.

International Agency for Research on Cancer. 1990. *IARC Monographs on the Evaluation of the Carcinogenic Risk of Chemicals to Humans: Pharmaceutical Drugs.* Vol. 50. Lyon, France: IARC.

Jagun, O., Ryan, M., and Waldron, H.A. 1982. "Urinary thioether excretion in nurses handling cytotoxic drugs." *Lancet* i:443-4.

Jeremic B, Shibamoto Y, Acimovic L, Milicic B, Milisavljevic S, Nikolic N, Aleksandrovic J, and Igrutinovic I. A randomized trial of three single-dose radiation therapy regimens in the treatment of metastatic bone pain. *International Journal of Radiation Oncology, Biology, Physics* 01 Aug 1998. 42:161-7. (1):

Johnson, E.G., and Janosik, J.E. 1989. "Manufacturers' recommendations for handling spilled antineoplastic agents." *Am. J. Hosp. Pharm.* 46:318-9.

Joint Commission on the Accreditation of Hospitals. 1986. *Accreditation Manual for Hospitals.* JCAH: Chicago.

Joishy SK and Walsh D. The opioid-sparing effects of intravenous ketorolac as an adjuvant analgesic in cancer pain: application in bone metastases and the opioid bowel syndrome. *Journal of Pain & Symptom Management* 1998. 16:334-9. (5):

Joranson D. Information about regulatory issues in pain

management. www.medsch.wisc.edu/painpolicy . June 1998.

Joranson DE, Ryan KM, Gilson AM, and Dahl JL. Trends in medical use and abuse of opioid analgesics. *JAMA* 05 Apr 2000. 283:1710-4. (13):

Juma, F.D., Rogers, H.J., Trounce, J.R., and Bradbrook, I.D. 1978. "Pharmacokinetics of intravenous cyclophosphamide in man, estimated by gas-liquid chromatography." *Cancer Chemother. Pharmacol.* 1:229-31.

Juni P, Witschi A, Bloch R, and Egger M. The hazards of scoring the quality of clinical trials for meta-analysis. *JAMA* 1999. 282:1054-60.

Kacmarek, R.M. 1990. "Ribavirin and pentamidine aerosols: Caregiver beware!" *Respiratory Care* 35:1034-6.

Kaiko RF, Kanner R, Foley KM, Wallenstein SL, Canel AM, Rogers AG, and Houde RW. Cocaine and morphine interaction in acute and chronic cancer pain. *Pain* Oct 1987. 31:35-45. (1):

Kalso E and Vainio A. Morphine and oxycodone hydrochloride in the management of cancer pain. *Clinical Pharmacology & Therapeutics* May 1990. 47:639-46. (5):

Kalso E, Heiskanen T, Rantio M, Rosenberg PH, and Vainio A. Epidural and subcutaneous morphine in the management of cancer pain: a double-blind cross-over study. *Pain* Oct 1996. 67:443-9. (2-3):

Kalso E, Tasmuth T, and Neuvonen P. Amitriptyline effectively relieves neuropathic pain following treatment of breast cancer. *Pain* Feb 1996. 64:293-302. (2):

Kalso E. Better standardisation will improve the quality of analgesic studies. *Acta Anaesthesiol Scand* 1996. 40:397-8.

Kane RL, Bernstein L, Wales J, and Rothenberg R. Hospice effectiveness in controlling pain. *JAMA* 10 May 1985. 253:2683-6. (18):

Kanner R. Diagnosis and management of pain in patients with cancer 10. Basel: Karger;. 1988. (Full Text in PMC)

Karakaya, A.E., Burgaz, S., and Bayhan, A. 1989. "The significance of urinary thioethers as indicators of exposure to alkylating agents." *Arch. Toxicol.* 13 (suppl.):117-9.

Kawamata M, Ishitani K, Ishikawa K, Sasaki H, Ota K, Omote K, and Namiki A. Comparison between celiac plexus block and morphine treatment on quality of life in patients with pancreatic cancer pain. *Pain* Mar 1996. 64:597-602. (3):

Kelson MC. Consumer collaboration, patient-defined outcomes and the preparation of Cochrane Reviews. 129-35. In Rice and Katz (eds) *Health Expectations.* London: Blackwell Science Ltd.; 1999. (Full Text in PMC)

Kilham, L. and Ferm, V.H. 1977. "Congenital anomalies induced in hamster embryos with ribavirin." *Science* 195:413-4.

Kleinberg, M.L. and Quinn, M.J. 1981. "Airborne drug levels in a laminar-flow hood."*Am. J. Hosp. Pharm.*38:1301-3.

Kolmodin-Hedman, B., Hartvig, P., Sorsa, M., and Falck, K. 1983. Occupational handling of cytostatic drugs. Arch. Toxicol.

Korte W, de Stoutz N, and Morant R. Day-to-day titration to initiate transdermal fentanyl in patients with cancer pain: short- and long-term experiences in a prospective study of 39 patients. *Journal of Pain & Symptom Management* Mar 1996. 11:139-46. (3):

Kravitz RL, Delafield JP, Hays RD, Drazin R, and Conolly M. Bedside charting of pain levels in hospitalized patients with cancer: a randomized controlled trial [see comments]. *Journal of Pain & Symptom Management* Feb 1996. 11:81-7. (2):

Kyle, R. A. 1984. "Second malignancies associated with chemotherapy." In Toxicity of Chemotherapy, Perry, M.C., and J.W. Yarbro (eds.), 479-506. Orlando: Grune & Stratton.

Kylmala T, Tammela T, Risteli L, Risteli J, Taube T, and Elomaa I. Evaluation of the effect of oral clodronate on skeletal metastases with type 1 collagen metabolites. A controlled trial of the Finnish Prostate Cancer Group. *European Journal of Cancer* 1993. 29A:821-5. (6):

Kylmala T, Taube T, Tammela TL, Risteli L, Risteli J, and Elomaa I. Concomitant i.v. and oral clodronate in the relief of bone pain—a double-blind placebo-controlled study in patients with prostate cancer. *British Journal of Cancer* 1997. 76:939-42. (7):

Labianca R, Pancera G, Aitini E, Barni S, Beretta A, Beretta GD, Cesana, Comella G, Cozzaglio L, and Cristoni M. Folinic acid + 5-fluorouracil (5-FU) versus equidose 5-FU in advanced colorectal cancer. Phase III study of 'GISCAD' (Italian Group for the Study of Digestive Tract Cancer). *Annals of Oncology* Oct 1991. 2:673-9. (9):

Lahtinen R, Laakso M, Palva I, Virkkunen P, and Elomaa I. Randomised, placebo-controlled multicentre trial of clodronate in multiple myeloma. *Lancet* 31 Oct 1992. 340:1049-52. [published erratum appears in *Lancet* 1992 Dec 5;340(8832):1420]. (8827):

Laidlaw, J.L., Connor, T.H., Theiss, J.C., et al. 1984. "Permeability of latex and polyvinyl chloride gloves to 20 antineoplastic drugs." *Am. J. Hosp. Pharm.* 41:2618-23.

Laidlaw, J.L., Connor, T.H., Theiss, J.C., et al. 1985. "Permeability of four disposable protective-clothing materials to seven antineoplastic drugs." *Am. J. Hosp. Pharm.* 42:2449-54.

Laird NM and Mosteller F. Some statistical methods for combining experimental results. *Int J Technol Assess Health Care* 1990. 6:5-30. (1):

Landis SH, Murray T, Bolden S, and Wingo PA. Cancer Statistics, 1999. *CA: A Cancer Journal for Clinicians* 1999. 49:8-11. (1):

Lang SS and Patt RB. You don't have to suffer. A complete guide to relieving cancer pain for patients and their families. New York: Oxford University Press;. 1994. (Full Text in PMC)

Larue F, Colleau SM, Brasseur L, and Cleeland CS. Multicentre study of cancer pain and its treatment in France [see comments]. *BMJ* 22 Apr 1995. 310:1034-7. (6986):

Lasagna L (ed). Combination drugs. Their use and regulation. New York: Stratton Intercontinental Medical Book Corp.; 1975. (Full Text in PMC)

Lasagna L, Mosteller F, von Felsinger JM, and Beecher HK. A study in placebo response. *American Journal of Medicine* Jun 1954. 770-9.

Lasch KE, Wilkes GM, Leonard C, Chew P, Montouri L, and Hilton SM. Using focus group methods to develop multicultural cancer pain education materials. Pain Management Nursing 2000. 1:129-138. (4): (PubMed)

Lau J, Ioannidis JP, and Schmid CH. Quantitative synthesis in systematic reviews. *Ann Intern Med* Nov 1997. 127:820-6. (9):

Lauretti GR, Reis MP, Mattos AL, Gomes JM, Oliveira AP, and Pereira NL. Epidural nonsteroidal antiinflammatory drugs for cancer pain. *Anesthesia & Analgesia* 1998. 86:117-8. (1):

Lee, S.B. 1988. "Ribavirin - Exposure to health care workers." *Am. Ind. Hyg. Assoc.* 49:A13-A14.

LeRoy, M.L., Roberts, M.J., and Theisen, J.A. 1983. "Procedures for handling antineoplastic injections in comprehensive cancer centers." *Am. Hosp Pharm.* 40:601-3.

Levick S, Jacobs C, Loukas DF, Gordon DH, Meyskens FL, and Uhm K. Naproxen sodium in treatment of bone pain due to metastatic cancer. *Pain* Dec 1988. 35:253-8. (3):

Lewington VJ, McEwan AJ, Ackery DM, Bayly RJ, Keeling DH, Macleod PM, Porter AT, and Zivanovic MA. A prospective, randomised double-blind crossover study to examine the efficacy of strontium-89 in pain palliation in patients with advanced prostate cancer metastatic to bone. *European Journal of Cancer* 1991. 27:954-8. (8):

Li QS, Cao SH, Xie GM, Gan YH, Ma HJ, Lu JZ, and Zhang ZH. Combined traditional Chinese medicine and Western medicine. Relieving effects of Chinese herbs, ear-acupuncture and epidural morphine on postoperative pain in liver cancer. *Chinese Medical Journal* Apr 1994. 107:289-94. (4):

Liew E and Hui YL. A preliminary study of long-term epidural morphine for cancer pain via a subcutaneously implanted reservoir. *Ma Tsui Hsueh Tsa Chi Anaesthesiologica Sinica* Mar 1989. 27:5-12. (1):

Lijmer JG, Mol BW, Heisterkamp S, Bonsel GJ, Prins MH, van der Meulen JH, and Bossuyt PM. Empirical evidence of design-related bias in studies of diagnostic tests [see comments]. *JAMA* 15 Sep 1999. 282:1061-6. (11):

Lillemoe KD, Cameron JL, Kaufman HS, Yeo CJ, Pitt HA, and Sauter PK. Chemical splanchnicectomy in patients with unresectable pancreatic cancer. A prospective randomized trial. *Ann Surg* May 1993. 217:447-57. (5):

Lipman AG, Jackson KC II, Tyler LS. Evidence-Based Symptom Control in Palliative Care. Binghamton NY:Haworth Press;. 2000. (Full Text in PMC)

Little M. Assignments of meaning in epidemiology. *Soc Sci Med* 1998. 47:1135-45. (9):

Loeser JD and Egan KJ (eds). Managing the chronic pain patient. Theory and practice at the University of Washington Multidisciplinary Pain Center. New York: Raven Press;. 1989. (Full Text in PMC)

Loeser JD. Evaluation of the pain patient. In Loeser JD, Butler SH, Chapman CR, Turk DC (eds). *Bonica's Management of Pain*, 3rd ed. Philadelphia:Lippincott, Williams & Wilkins;. 2001. 265-266. (Full Text in PMC)

Lunn, G. and Sansone, E.B. 1989. "Validated methods for handling spilled antineoplastic agents." *Am. J. Hosp. Pharm.* 46:1131.

Lunn, G., Sansone, E.B., Andrews, A.W., and Hellwig, L.C. 1989. "Degradation and disposal of some antineoplastic drugs." *J. Pharm. Sciences* 78:652-9.

Macbeth FR, Bolger JJ, Hopwood P, Bleehen NM, Cartmell J, Girling DJ, Machin D, Stephens RJ, and Bailey AJ. Randomized trial of palliative two-fraction versus more intensive 13-fraction radiotherapy for patients with inoperable non-small cell lung cancer and good performance status. Medical Research Council Lung Cancer Working Party [see comments]. *Clinical Oncology (Royal College of Radiologists)* 1996. 8:167-75. (3):

Macrae WA and Bavies HTO. Chronic postsurgical pain. In Crombie IK, Croft PR, Linton SJ, LeResche L, and von Korff M (eds). *Epidemiology of Pain.* Seattle: IASP Press;. 1999. 125-42. (Full Text in PMC)

Madrid JL, Fatela LV, Alcorta J, Guillen F, and Lobato RD. Intermittent intrathecal morphine by means of an implantable reservoir: a survey of 100 cases. *Journal of Pain & Symptom Management* 1988. 3:67-71. (2):

Madsen EL. Painful bone metastasis: efficacy of radiotherapy assessed by the patients: a randomized trial comparing 4 Gy X 6 versus 10 Gy X 2. *International Journal of Radiation Oncology, Biology, Physics* Dec 1983. 9:1775-9. (12):

Mant D. Can randomised trials inform clinical decisions about individual patients? *Lancet* 27 Feb 1999. 353:743-6. (9154):

Mark DH and Glass RM. Impact of new technologies in medicine: a global theme issue [editorial]. *JAMA* 17 Nov 1999. 282:-. (19):

Martino G, Emanueli A, Mandelli V, and Ventafridda V. A controlled study of the analgetic effect of two non-steroidal anti-inflammatory drugs in cancer pain. *Arzneimittel-Forschung* 1978. 28:1657-9. (9):

Martino G, Ventafridda V, Parini J, and Emanueli A. A controlled study on the analgesic activity of indoprofen in patients with cancer pain. [Monograph] In Bonica JJ and Albe-Fessard D eds. *Pharmacological Agents in*

Chronic Pain, Advances in Pain Research and Therapy, Vol 1:New York: Raven Press;. 1976. 573-8.

Martoni A, Guaraldi M, Camera P, Biagi R, Marri S, Beghe F, and Pannuti F. Controlled clinical study on the use of dichloromethylene diphosphonate in patients with breast carcinoma metastasizing to the skeleton. *Oncology* 1991. 48:97-101. (2):

Matthews, T. and Boehme, R. 1988. "Antiviral activity and mechanism of action of ganciclovir." *Rev. Infect. Diseases* 10(suppl 3):s490-94.

Max M. Methodological issues in the design of analgesic clinical trials. In Max M (ed). *Pain 1999 - An updated review: Refresher course syllabus.* Seattle: IASP Press;. 1999. 6:299-308.

Max MB and Portenoy RK. Pain research: designing clinical trials in palliative care. *Oxford textbook of palliative medicine 2nd ed.* New York: Oxford University Press, Inc.; 1998. 167-178. (Full Text in PMC)

Max MB. Thirteen consecutive well-designed randomized trials show that antidepressants reduce pain in diabetic neuropathy and postherpetic neuralgia. *Pain Forum* 1995. 4:248-53. (4):

McCaffery M and Pasero C. Pain clinical manual. 2nd ed. St. Louis: Mosby, Inc.; 1999. (Full Text in PMC)

McCloskey EV, MacLennan IC, Drayson MT, Chapman C, Dunn J, and Kanis JA. A randomized trial of the effect of clodronate on skeletal morbidity in multiple myeloma. MRC Working Party on Leukaemia in Adults. *British Journal of Haematology* Feb 1998. 100:317-25. (2):

McCorkle R, Benoliel JQ, Donaldson G, Georgiadou F, Moinpour C, and Goodell. A randomized clinical trial of home nursing care for lung cancer patients. *Cancer* 15 Sep 1989. 64:1375-82. (6):

McDevitt, J.J., Lees, P.S.J., and McDiarmid, M.A. 1993. "Exposure of Hospital Pharmacists and Nurses to Antineoplastic Agents." *J. Occup. Med.* 35:57-60.

McDiarmid, M.A. and Emmett, E.A. 1987. "Biological monitoring and medical surveillance of workers exposed to antineoplastic agents." *Seminars in Occup. Med.* 2:109-17.

McDiarmid, M.A., and Jacobson-Kram, D. 1989. "Aerosolized pentamidine and public health." *Lancet* ii:863-864.

McDiarmid, M.A., Egan, T., Furio, M., et al. 1988. "Sampling for airborne fluorouracil in a hospital drug preparation area." *Am. J. Hosp. Pharm.* 43:1942-5.

McDiarmid, M.A., Gurley, H. T., and Arrington, D. 1991. "Pharmaceuticals as hospital hazards: Managing the risks." *J. Occup. Med.* 33:155-8.

McDiarmid, M.A., Kolodner, K., Humphrey, F., et al. 1992. "Baseline and phosphoramide mustard-induced sister-chromatid exchanges in pharmacists handling anticancer drugs." *Mutation Research* 279:199-204.

McDiarmid, M.A., Schaefer, J., Richard, C.L., Chaisson, R.E., and Tepper, B.S. 1992. "Efficacy of engineering controls in reducing occupational exposure to aerosolized pentamidine." *Chest* 102:1764-6.

McEvoy, G. K., ed. 1993. *American Hospital Formulary Service Drug Information.* Bethesda: American Society of Hospital Pharmacists.

McLendon, B.F. and Bron, A.F. 1978. "Corneal toxicity from vinblastine solution." *Br. J. Ophthalmol.* 62;97-9.

McQuay H and Moore A. An evidence-based resource for pain relief. Oxford: Oxford University Press;. 1998. (Full Text in PMC)

McQuay H, Carroll D, Jadad AR, Wiffen P, and Moore A.

Anticonvulsant drugs for management of pain: a systematic review. *BMJ* 21 Oct 1995. 311:1047-52. (7012):

McQuay H. Opioids in pain management. *Lancet* 1999. 353:2229-33. (9171):

McQuay HJ, Carroll D, and Moore RA. Radiotherapy for painful bone metastases: a systematic review. *Clinical Oncology* (Royal College of Radiologists) 1997. 9:150-4. (3):

McQuay HJ, Tramer M, Nye BA, Carroll D, Wiffen PJ, and Moore RA. A systematic review of antidepressants in neuropathic pain [see comments]. *Pain* Dec 1996. 68:217-27. (2-3):

Medical Research Council (MRC) randomised trial of palliative radiotherapy with two fractions or a single fraction in patients with inoperable non-small-cell lung cancer (NSCLC) and poor performance status. *British Journal of Cancer* Jun 1992. 65:934-41. (6):

Meglio M and Cioni B. The role of percutaneous cordotomy in the treatment of chronic cancer pain. *Acta Neurochir* (Wien) 1981. 59:111-21. (1-2):

Mercadante S, Armata M, and Salvaggio L. Pain characteristics of advanced lung cancer patients referred to a palliative care service. *Pain* Oct 1994. 59:141-5. (1):

Mercadante S, Casuccio A, Agnello A, Pumo S, Kargar J, and Garofalo S. Analgesic effects of nonsteroidal anti-inflammatory drugs in cancer pain due to somatic or visceral mechanisms. *Journal of Pain & Symptom Management* May 1999. 17:351-6. (5):

Mercadante S, Maddaloni S, Roccella S, and Salvaggio L. Predictive factors in advanced cancer pain treated only by analgesics. *Pain* 1992. 50:151-5. (2):

Mercadante S, Salvaggio L, Dardanoni G, Agnello A, and Garofalo S. Dextropropoxyphene versus morphine in opioid-naive cancer patients with pain. *Journal of Pain & Symptom Management* Feb 1998. 15:76-81. (2):

Mercadante S, Sapio M, Caligara M, Serretta R, Dardanoni G, and Barresi L. Opioid-sparing effect of diclofenac in cancer pain. *Journal of Pain & Symptom Management* 1997. 14:15-20. (1):

Mercadante S. Celiac plexus block versus analgesics in pancreatic cancer pain. *Pain* 1993. 52:187-92.

Mercadante S. Pain treatment and outcomes for patients with advanced cancer who receive follow-up care at home [see comments]. *Cancer* 15 Apr 1999a. 85:1849-58. (8):

Mercadante S. World Health Organization Guidelines: problem areas in cancer pain management. *Cancer Control: Journal of the Moffitt Cancer Center* 1999b. 6:191-7. (2):

Merskey H and Bogduk N (eds). Classification of chronic pain. Description of chronic pain syndromes and definitions of pain terms. 2nd ed. Seattle: IASP Press;. 1994. (Full Text in PMC)

Meuret G and Jocham H. Patient-controlled analgesia (PCA) in the domiciliary care of tumour patients. *Cancer Treatment Reviews* Jan 1996. 22:137-40. (Supplement A):

Meyers CA. Neurocognitive dysfunction in cancer patients. *Oncology* Jan 2000. 14:75-9. (1):

Miaskowski C and Levine JD. Does opioid analgesia show a gender preference for females? *Pain Forum* 1999. 8:34-44.

Miaskowski C. Pain Management: quality assurance and

changing practice. In Gebhart G, Hammond D, and Jensen TS (eds). *Proceedings of the* 7rd *World Congress of Pain*. Seattle: IASP Press;. 1994. 75-96.

Mignault GG, Latreille J, Viguie F, Richer P, Lemire F, Harsanyi Z, and Stewart JH. Control of cancer-related pain with MS Contin: a comparison between 12-hourly and 8-hourly administration [see comments]. *Journal of Pain & Symptom Management* Aug 1995. 10:416-22. (6):

Miller AB (ed.). The World Health Organisation Global Programme for Cancer Control. National Cancer Control Programmes. Policies and managerial guidelines. Geneva: World Health Organisation;. 1993. (Full Text in PMC)

Miller AB, Hoogstraten B, Staquet M, and Winkler A. Reporting results of cancer treatment. *Cancer* 01 Jan 1981. 47:207-14. (1):

Miller, B.M. et al. 1986. *Laboratory Safety Principles and Practices*. American Society for Microbiology: Washington D.C.

Minotti V, Betti M, Ciccarese G, Fumi G, Tonato M, and Del Favero A. A double-blind study comparing two single-dose regimens of ketorolac with diclofenac in pain due to cancer. *Pharmacotherapy* May 1998a. 18:504-8. (3):

Minotti V, De Angelis V, Righetti E, Celani MG, Rossetti R, Lupatelli M, Tonato M, Pisati R, Monza G, Fumi G, and Del Favero A. Double-blind evaluation of short-term analgesic efficacy of orally administered diclofenac, diclofenac plus codeine, and diclofenac plus imipramine in chronic cancer pain. *Pain* Feb 1998b. 74:133-7. (2-3):

Minotti V, Patoia L, Roila F, Basurto C, Tonato M, Pasqualucci V, Maresca V, and Del Favero A. Double-blind evaluation of analgesic efficacy of orally administered diclofenac, nefopam, and acetylsalicylic acid (ASA) plus codeine in chronic cancer pain. *Pain* Feb 1989. 36:177-83. (2):

Miser AW, Dothage JA, Wesley RA, and Miser JS. The prevalence of pain in a pediatric and young adult cancer population. *Pain* Apr 1987. 29:73-83. (1):

Miser AW, McCalla J, Dothage JA, Wesley M, and Miser JS. Pain as a presenting symptom in children and young adults with newly diagnosed malignancy. *Pain* Apr 1987. 29:85-90. (1):

Mitchell JD. Global populations growing older. In Brown L, Renner M, Flavin C, Starke L et al., (eds). *Vital signs 1997. The environmental trends that are shaping our future.* New York: W.W. Norton;. 1997. 124-5. (Full Text in PMC)

Modell W. Relief of symptoms. 2nd ed. St. Louis: CV Mosby Company;. 1961. (Full Text in PMC)

Moertel CG, Ahmann DL, Taylor WF, and Schwartau N. Relief of pain by oral medications. A controlled evaluation of analgesic combinations. *JAMA* 01 Jul 1974. 229:55-9. (1):

Mogil JS. The genetic mediation of individual differences in sensitivity to pain and its inhibition. *Proceedings of the National Academy of Sciences, USA* 1999. 96:7744-51.

Moher D, Dulberg CS, Wells GA. Statistical power, sample size, and their reporting in randomized controlled trials. *JAMA*. 1994. 272:122-4. (PubMed)

Moher D, Jadad AR, Nichol G, Penman M, Tugwell P, and Walsh S. Assessing the quality of randomized controlled trials: an annotated bibliography of scales and checklists. *Control Clin Trials* Feb 1995. 16:62-73. (1):

Moore R and Brodsgaard I. Cross-cultural investigations of pain. Crombie I (ed). *Epidemiology of pain.* Seattle: IASP Press;. 1999. 53-80.

Moore RA, Gavaghan D, Tramer MR, Collins SL, and McQuay HJ. Size is everything—large amounts of information are needed to overcome random effects in estimating direction and magnitude of treatment effects. *Pain* Dec 1998. 78:209-16. (3):

Morley JS. New perspectives in our use of opioids. *Pain Forum* 1999. 8:200-5. (4):

Morris DB. Illness and culture in the postmodern age. Berkeley: University of California Press; 1998.

Moulin DE, Johnson NG, Murray-Parsons N, Geoghegan MF, Goodwin VA, and Chester MA. Subcutaneous narcotic infusions for cancer pain: treatment outcome and guidelines for use. *CMAJ* Mar 1992. 146:891-7. (6):

Moulin DE, Kreeft JH, Murray-Parsons N, and Bouquillon AI. Comparison of continuous subcutaneous and intravenous hydromorphone infusions for management of cancer pain. *Lancet* 23 Feb 1991. 337:465-8. (8739):

Mulrow C and Cook D. Systematic reviews. Synthesis of best evidence for health care decisions. Philadelphia: American College of Physicians;. 1998. (Full Text in PMC)

Mulrow CD and Oxman AD (eds). Cochrane collaboration handbook [updated September 1997]. How to conduct a cochrane systematic review. In The Cochrane Library [database on disk and CDROM]. Issue 4. Oxford: Update Software;. 1997. (Full Text in PMC)

Myers KG and Trotman IF. Use of ketorolac by continuous subcutaneous infusion for the control of cancer-related pain. *Postgraduate Medical Journal* May 1994. 70:359-62. (823):

Myles PS. Why we need large randomized studies in anaesthesia. *Br J Anaesth* Dec 1999. 83:833-4. (6):

Nagaro T, Amakawa K, Yamauchi Y, Tabo E, Kimura S, and Arai T. Percutaneous cervical cordotomy and subarachnoid phenol block using fluoroscopy in pain control of costopleural syndrome. *Pain* Sep 1994. 58:325-30. (3):

National Council for Radiation Protection and Measurements (NCRP). 1978. *Radiation Protection for Medical and Allied Health Personnel.* NCRP Report #48. NCRP: Washington, DC.

National Fire Protection Association (NFPA). 1987. *Health Care Facilities Handbook.* 2nd ed. NFPA: Quincy, MA.

National Institute for Occupational Safety and Health (NIOSH). 1977. *Criteria for a Recommended Standard: Occupational Exposure to Waste Anesthetic Gases and Vapors.* DHEW: NIOSH Publication No. 77-140. NIOSH: Cincinnati, OH.

National Institute for Occupational Safety and Health (NIOSH). 1988. *Guidelines for Protecting the Safety and Health of Health Care Workers.* DHHS: NIOSH Publication No. 88-119. NIOSH: Cincinnati, OH.

National Institute for Occupational Safety and Health (NIOSH). 1989. *Ethylene Oxide Sterilizers in Health Care Facilities: Engineering Controls and Work Practices.* DHHS: NIOSH Publication No. 89-116. July 13, 1989. NIOSH: Cincinnati, OH.

National Institute for Occupational Safety and Health (NIOSH). 1977. *Criteria for a Recommended Standard: Occupational Exposure to Waste Anesthetic Gases and Vapors.* DHEW: NIOSH Publication No. 77-140. NIOSH: Cincinnati, OH.

National Institute for Occupational Safety and Health (NIOSH). 1988. *Guidelines for Protecting the Safety and Health of Health Care Workers.* DHHS: NIOSH Publication No. 88-119. NIOSH: Cincinnati, OH.

National Institute for Occupational Safety and Health (NIOSH). 1989. *Ethylene Oxide Sterilizers in Health Care Facilities: Engineering Controls and Work Practices.* DHHS: NIOSH Publication No. 89-116. July 13, 1989. NIOSH: Cincinnati, OH.

National Sanitation Foundation. 1990. *Standard No. 49 for Class II (Laminar Flow) Biohazard Cabinetry.* Ann Arbor: National Sanitation Foundation.

National Study Commission on Cytotoxic Exposure. 1983. *Recommendations for Handling Cytotoxic Agents.* Louis P. Jeffrey, Sc.D., Chairman, Rhode Island Hospital, Providence, Rhode Island.

Neal, A.D., Wadden, R.A., and Chiou, W. L. 1983. "Exposure of hospital workers to airborne antineoplastic agents." *Am. J. Hosp. Pharm.* 40:597-601.

Nguyen, T.V., Theiss, J.C., and Matney, T.S. "Exposure of pharmacy personnel to mutagenic antineoplastic drugs." *Cancer Research* 42:4792-6.

Nielsen OS, Bentzen SM, Sandberg E, Gadeberg CC, and Timothy AR. Randomized trial of single dose versus fractionated palliative radiotherapy of bone metastases. *Radiotherapy & Oncology* Jun 1998. 47:233-40. (3):

Niewald M, Tkocz HJ, Abel U, Scheib T, Walter K, Nieder C, Schnabel K, Berberich W, Kubale R, and Fuchs M. Rapid course radiation therapy vs. more standard treatment: a randomized trial for bone metastases. *International Journal of Radiation Oncology, Biology, Physics* 01 Dec 1996. 36:1085-9. (5):

Nikula E., Kiviniitty K., Leisti J., and Taskinen, P. "Chromosome aberrations in lymphocytes of nurses handling cytostatic agents." *Scand. J. Work Environ. Health.* 1984;10:71-4.

Nitescu P, Sjoberg M, Appelgren L, and Curelaru I. Complications of intrathecal opioids and bupivacaine in the treatment of "refractory" cancer pain. *Clinical Journal of Pain* Mar 1995. 11:45-62. (1):

Norppa, H., Sorsa, M., Vainio, H., et al. 1980. "Increased sister chromatid exchange frequencies in lymphocytes of nurses handling cytostatic drugs." *Scand. J. Work Envir. Health* 6:299-301.

O'Brien T, Mortimer PG, McDonald CJ, and Miller AJ. A randomized crossover study comparing the efficacy and tolerability of a novel once-daily morphine preparation (MXL capsules) with MST Continus tablets in cancer patients with severe pain. *Palliative Medicine* Nov 1997. 11:475-82. (6):

O'Rourke N, McCloskey E, Houghton F, Huss H, and Kanis JA. Double-blind, placebo-controlled, dose-response trial of oral clodronate in patients with bone metastases. *Journal of Clinical Oncology* Apr 1995. 13:929-34. (4):

Occupational Safety and Health Administration (OSHA). 1986. *Guidelines for Antineoplastic (Cytotoxic) Drugs.* OSHA: Washington, DC.

Occupational Safety and Health Administration (OSHA). 1987. *Chemical Information Manual.* U.S. Government Printing Office: Washington, DC.

Occupational Safety and Health Administration (OSHA). 1989. *Enforcement Procedures for Occupational Exposure to Hepatitis B Virus (HBV) and Human Immunodeficiency Virus (HIV).* OSHA: Washington, DC.

Okawa T, Kita M, Goto M, Nishijima H, and Miyaji N. Randomized prospective clinical study of small, large and twice-a-day fraction radiotherapy for painful bone metastases. *Radiotherapy & Oncology* Oct 1988. 13:99-104. (2):

Osterweis M, Kleinman A, and Mechanic D. Pain and disability: Clinical, behavioral, and public policy perspectives. Committee of Pain Disability and Chronic Illness Behavior. Institute of Medicine. Washington, DC: National Academy Press;. 1987. (Full Text in PMC)

Oyama T, Jin T, Yamaya R, Ling N, and Guillemin R. Profound analgesic effects of beta-endorphin in man. *Lancet* Jan 1980. 1:122-4. (8160):

Pain assessment and management standards. In *Comprehensive accreditation manual for hospitals: the official handbook.* Oakbrook: The Commission;. 2000. (Full Text in PMC)

Palmer, R.G., Dore, C.J., and Denman, A.M. 1984. "Chlorambucil-induced chromosome damage to human lymphocytes is dose-dependent and cumulative." *Lancet* i:246-9.

Panich A and Charnvej L. Comparison of morphine slow release tablet (MST) and morphine sulphate solution (MSS) in the treatment of cancer pain. *Journal of the Medical Association of Thailand* Dec 1993. 76:672-6. (12):

Papo I and Visca A. Phenol rhizotomy in the treatment of cancer pain. *Anesth Analg* 1974. 53:993-7. (6):

Parris WCV. Cancer pain management: principles and practice. Boston: Butterworth-Heinemann; 1997.

Pasqualucci V, Tantucci C, Paoletti F, Dottorini ML, Bifarini G, Belfiori R, Berioli MB, Grassi V, and Sorbini CA.

Buprenorphine vs. morphine via the epidural route: a controlled comparative clinical study of respiratory effects and analgesic activity. *Pain* Jun 1987. 29:273-86. (3):

Paterson AH, Powles TJ, Kanis JA, McCloskey E, Hanson J, and Ashley S. Double-blind controlled trial of oral clodronate in patients with bone metastases from breast cancer. *Journal of Clinical Oncology* Jan 1993. 11:59-65. (1):

Patt RB. Cancer pain. Philadelphia: JB Lippincott Company;. 1993. (Full Text in PMC)

Patterson, W. et al. 1985. *Occupational Hazards to Hospital Personnel.* Annals of Internal Medicine. 102:658-680.

Payne R and Gonzales G. Pathophysiology of pain in cancer and other terminal diseases. In Doyle D, Hanks G, MacDonald N (eds). *Oxford textbook of palliative medicine.* New York: Oxford University Press, Inc.; 1999. 299-309. (Full Text in PMC)

Payne R, Patt RB, and Hill CS. Assessment and treatment of cancer pain 12. Seattle: IASP Press;. 1998. (Full Text in PMC)

Pellegrini A, Massidda B, Pellegrini P, Defraia E, Usai A, Parrinello L, Bruni G, Rigamonti G, and Sacchetti G. Effect of i.v. indoprofen on cancer pain and serum prolactin and growth hormone levels - a controlled pharmocologic study vs i.m. morphine and placebo. *Int J Clin Pharmacol Ther Toxicol* Sep 1983. 21:483-6. (9):

Perkins FM and Kehlet H. Chronic pain as an outcome of surgery. A review of predictive factors. *Anesthesiology.* 2000. 93:1123-33. (4):

Physician's Desk Reference. 1991. Physician's Desk Reference. 45th ed. Page 730. Barnhart, E.R., pub. Oradell, New Jersey: Medical Economics Data.

Plummer JL, Cherry DA, Cousins MJ, Gourlay GK. Onley MM, and Evans KH. Long-term spinal administration of morphine in cancer and non-cancer pain: a retrospective study. *Pain* Mar 1991. 44:215-20. (3):

Pocock SJ. Clinical trials: a practical approach. New York: John Wiley & Sons;. 1998. (Full Text in PMC)

Pohlova, H., Cerna, M., and Rossner, P. 1986. "Chromosomal aberrations, SCE and urine mutagenicity in workers occupationally exposed to cytostatic drugs." *Mutation Res.* 174:213-7.

Polati E, Finco G, Gottin L, Bassi C, Pederzoli P, and Ischia S. Prospective randomized double-blind trial of neurolytic coeliac plexus block in patients with pancreatic cancer. *Br J Surg* Feb 1998. 85:199-201. (2):

Portenoy RK and Hagen NA. Breakthrough pain: definition, prevalence and characteristics [see comments]. *Pain* Jun 1990. 41:273-81. (3):

Portenoy RK and Lesage P. Management of cancer pain. *Lancet* 1999. 353:1695-700.

Portenoy RK, Maldonado M, Fitzmartin R, Kaiko RF, and Kanner R. Oral controlled-release morphine sulfate. Analgesic efficacy and side effects of a 100-mg tablet in cancer pain patients. *Cancer* 01 Jun 1989. 63:2284-8. (11 Suppl):

Porter AT, McEwan AJ, Powe JE, Reid R, McGowan DG, Lukka H, Sathyanarayana JR, Yakemchuk VN, Thomas GM, and Erlich LE. Results of a randomized phase-III trial to evaluate the efficacy of strontium-89 adjuvant to local field external beam irradiation in the management of endocrine resistant metastatic prostate cancer. *International Journal of Radiation Oncology, Biology, Physics* 02 Apr 1993. 25:805-13. (5):

Price P, Hoskin PJ, Easton D, Austin D, Palmer SG, and Yarnold JR. Prospective randomised trial of single and multifraction radiotherapy schedules in the treatment of painful bony metastases. *Radiotherapy & Oncology* Aug 1986. 6:247-55. (4):

Pud D, Eisenberg E, Spitzer A, Adler R, Fried G, and Yarnitsky D. The NMDA receptor antagonist amantadine reduces surgical neuropathic pain in cancer patients: a double blind, randomized, placebo controlled trial. *Pain* Apr 1998. 75:349-54. (2-3):

Puglisi G and Garagiola U. Pirprofen and Pentazocine in the treatment of cancer pain. *Current Therapeutic Research* March 1989. 45:333-338. (3):

Pyy, L., Sorsa, M., and Hakala, E. 1988. "Ambient monitoring of cyclophosphamide in manufacture and hospitals." *Am. Ind. Hyg. Assoc. J.* 49:314-7.

Quilty PM, Kirk D, Bolger JJ, Dearnaley DP, Lewington VJ, Mason MD, Reed NS, Russell JM, and Yardley J. A comparison of the palliative effects of strontium-89 and external beam radiotherapy in metastatic prostate cancer. *Radiotherapy & Oncology* Apr 1994. 31:33-40. (1):

Quinn SF, Murtagh FR, Chatfield R, and Kori SH. CT-guided nerve root block and ablation. *Am J Roentgenol* Dec 1988. 151:1213-6. (6):

Raj PP. The practical management of pain. 2nd ed. St. Louis: Mosby Year Book;. 1992. (Full Text in PMC)

Ramesh PR, Kumar KS, Rajagopal MR, Balachandran P, and Warrier PK. Managing morphine-induced constipation: a controlled comparison of an Ayurvedic formulation and senna. *Journal of Pain & Symptom Management* Oct 1998. 16:240-4. (4):

Rees GJ, Devrell CE, Barley VL, and Newman HF. Palliative

radiotherapy for lung cancer: two versus five fractions. *Clinical Oncology* (Royal College of Radiologists) 1997. 9:90-5. (2):

Reich, S.D. and Bachur, N.R. 1975. "Contact dermatitis associated with adriamycin (NSC-123127) and daunorubicin (NSC-82151)." *Cancer Chemotherap. Reports* 59:677-8.

Resche I, Chatal JF, Pecking A, Ell P, Duchesne G, Rubens R, Fogelman, Houston S, Fauser A, Fischer M, and Wilkins D. A dose-controlled study of 153Sm-ethylenediaminetetramethylenephosphonate (EDTMP) in the treatment of patients with painful bone metastases. *European Journal of Cancer* Sep 1997. 33:1583-91. (10):

Reynolds, R.D., Ignoffo, R., Lawrence, J., et al. 1982. "Adverse reactions to AMSA in medical personnel." *Cancer Treat. Rep.* 66:1885.

Richmond, J. 1988. *Safe Practices and Procedures for Working with Human Specimens in Biomedical Research Laboratories.* Journal of Clinical Immunoassay 11(3): 115-119.

Rizzo M, Mazzei T, Mini E, Bartoletti R, and Periti P. Leuprorelin acetate depot in advanced prostatic cancer: a phase II multicentre trial. *Journal of International Medical Research* 1990. 18:114-25. (Suppl 1):

Robertson AG, Reed NS, and Ralston SH. Effect of oral clodronate on metastatic bone pain: a double-blind, placebo-controlled study. *Journal of Clinical Oncology* Sep 1995. 13:2427-30. (9):

Roca G, Aguilar JL, Gomar C, Mazo V, Costa J, and Vidal F. Nimodipine fails to enhance the analgesic effect of slow release morphine in the early phases of cancer pain treatment. *Pain* Dec 1996. 68:239-43. (2-3):

Rodriguez M, Barutell C, Rull M, Galvez R, Pallares J, Vidal F, Aliaga, Moreno J, Puerta J, and Ortiz P. Efficacy and tolerance of oral dipyrone versus oral morphine for cancer pain. *European Journal of Cancer* 1994. 30A:584-7. (5):

Rogers, B. 1987. "Health hazards to personnel handling antineoplastic agents." *Occupational Medicine: State of the Art Reviews* 2:513-24.

Rogers, B. and Emmett, E.A. 1987. "Handling antineoplastic agents: Urine mutagenicity in nurses." *IMAGE Journal of Nursing Scholarship.* 19:108-113

Rose, S.L. 1984. *Clinical Laboratory Safety.* J.B. Lippincott Co.: Philadelphia, PA.

Rosner, F. 1976. "Acute leukemia as a delayed consequence of cancer chemotherapy." *Cancer*37:1033-6.

Rosser WW. Application of evidence from randomised controlled trials to general practice. *Lancet* 20 Feb 1999. 353:661-4. (9153):

Roth A and Kolaric K. Analgetic activity of calcitonin in patients with painful osteolytic metastases of breast cancer. Results of a controlled randomized study. *Oncology* 1986. 43:283-7. (5):

Rothbard MJ, Kotsilimbas DG, Jacobson SA, and Sall S. Relief of intractable pain in cervical carcinoma with percutaneous radiofrequency cordotomy. *Obstet Gynecol* Jul 1972. 40:50-5. (1):

Rothman KJ and Michels KB. The continuing unethical use of placebo controls. *N Engl J Med* 11 Aug 1994. 331:394-8. (6):

Rudolph, R., Suzuki, M., and Luce, J. K. 1979. "Experimental skin necrosis produced by adriamycin." *Cancer Treat. Reports* 63:529-37.

Sacchetti G, Camera P, Rossi AP, Martioni A, Bruni G, and Pannuti F. Injectable ketoprofen vs. acetylsalicylic acid for the relief of severe cancer pain: a double-blind, crossover trial. *Drug Intelligence & Clinical Pharmacy* May 1984. 18:403-6.

Sackett DL, Richardson SW, Rosenberg W, and Haynes RB. Evidence-based medicine. How to practice & teach EBM. New York: Churchill Livingsone;. 1997. (Full Text in PMC)

Schafer, A.L. 1981. "Teratogenic effects of antileukemic therapy." *Arch. Int. Med.* 141:514-5.

Selevan, S.G., Lindbolm, M.L., Hornung, R.W., and Hemminki, K. 1985. "A study of occupational exposure to antineoplastic drugs and fetal loss in nurses." *New England J. Med.* 313:1173-8.

Sieber, S.M. 1975. "Cancer chemotherapeutic agents and carcinogenesis." *Cancer Chemotherap. Reports* 59:915-8.

Sieber, S.M., and Adamson, R.H. 1975. "Toxicity of antineoplastic agents in man: Chromosomal aberrations, antifertility effects, congenital malformations, and carcinogenic potential." *Adv. Cancer Res.* 22:57-155.

Siebert, D. and Simon, U. 1973. "Cyclophosphamide: Pilot study of genetically active metabolites in the urine of a treated human patient." *Mutat. Res.* 19:65-72.

Slevin, M.L., Ang, L.M., Johnston, A., and Turner, P. 1984. "The efficiency of protective gloves used in the handling of cytotoxic drugs." *Cancer Chemo. Pharmacol.* 12:151-3.

Smaldone, G.C., Vincicuerra, C., and Marchese, J. 1991. "Detection of inhaled pentamidine in health care workers." *New England J. Med.* 325:891-2.

Sommargren, C.E. (ed.). 1989. *AACN Handbook on Occupational Hazards for the Critical Care Nurse.* American Association of Critical-Care Nurses, Occupational Hazards Task Force. AACN: Chicago, IL.

Sorsa, M., Hemminki, K., and Vanio, H. 1985. "Occupational exposure to anticancer drugs — Potential and real hazards." *Mut. Res.* 154:135-49.

Sotaniemi, E.A., Sutinen, S., Arranto, A.J., et al. 1983. "Liver damage in nurses handling cytostatic agents."*Acta Med. Scand.* 214:181-9.

Stellman, J.M. 1987. "The spread of chemotherapeutic agents at work: Assessment through stimulation." *Cancer Investigation* 5:75-81.

Stephens, J.D., Golbus, M.S., Miller, T. R., et al. 1980. "Multiple congenital abnormalities in a fetus exposed to 5-fluorouracil during the first trimester." *Am. J. Obstet. Gynecol.* 137:747-9.

Stiller, A., Obe, G., Bool, I., and Pribilla, W. 1983. "No elevation of the frequencies of chromosomal aberrations as a consequence of handling cytostatic drugs." *Mut. Res.* 121:253-9.

Stoikes, M.E., Carlson, J.D., Farris, F.F., and Walker, P.R. 1987. "Permeability of latex and polyvinyl chloride gloves to fluorouracil and methotrexate." *Am. J. Hosp. Pharm.* 44:1341-6.

Stucker, I., Caillard, J.F., Collin, R., et al. 1990. "Risk of spontaneous abortion among nurses handling antineoplastic drugs." *Scand. J. Work Environ. Health* 16:102-7.

Stucker, I., Hirsch, A., Doloy, T., et al. 1986. "Urine mutagenicity, chromosomal abnormalities and sister chromatid exchanges in lymphocytes of nurses handling cytostatic drugs." *Int. Arch. Occup. Environ. Health* 57:195-205.

Texas Hospital Association (THA) and Shared Hospital Electrical Safety Services. 1973. *Electrical Safety Guide.* THA: Austin.

U.S. Department of Health and Human Services. Public Health Service. National Institutes of Health. 1992. *Recommendations for the Safe Handling of Cytotoxic Drugs.* NIH Publication No. 92-2621.

U.S. Department of Labor, Occupational Safety and Health Administration. 1984. Respiratory Protection Standard. 29 CFR 1910.134.

U.S. Department of Labor, Occupational Safety and Health Administration. 1986. *Work practice guidelines for personnel dealing with cytotoxic (antineoplastic) drugs.* OSHA Publication #8-1.1.

U.S. Department of Labor, Occupational Safety and Health Administration. 1991. Occupational Exposure to Bloodborne Pathogens Standard. 29 CFR 1910.1030.

United States Department of Health and Human Services. 1988. *Biosafety in Microbiological and Biomedical Laboratories.* HHS: Washington, DC.

Vaccari, F.L., Tonat, K., DeChristoforo, R., et al. 1984. "Disposal of antineoplastic wastes at the NIH." *Am. J. Hosp. Pharm.* 41:87-92.

Valanis, B., Vollmer, W.M., Labuhn, K., Glass, A., and Corelle, C. 1992. "Antineoplastic drug handling protection after OSHA guidelines: Comparison by profession, handling activity, and worksite." *J. Occup. Med.* 34:149-55.

Vesley, D., Hartman, M.S., and Heidi, M. 1988. *Laboratory Acquired Infections and Injuries in Clinical Laboratories:*

A 1986 Survey. American Journal of Public Health 78(9):1213-1215. Benhamou, S., Pot-Deprun, J., Sancho-Garnier, H., and Chouroulinkov, I. 1988. "Sister chromatid exchanges and chromosomal aberrations in lymphocytes of nurses handling cytostatic drugs." I 41:350-3.

Waksvik, H., Klepp, O., and Brogger, A. 1981. "Chromosome analyses of nurses handling cytostatic agents." *Cancer Treat. Reports* 65:607-10.

Wall, R.L. and Clausen, K.P. 1975. "Carcinoma of the urinary bladder in patients receiving cyclophosphamide." *New England J. Med.* 293:271-3.

Weisburger, J.H., Griswold, D.P., Prejean J.D., et al. 1975. "Tumor induction by cytostatics. The carcinogenic properties of some of the principal drugs used in clinical cancer chemotherapy." *Recent Results Cancer Res.* 52:1-17.

Zimmerman, P.F., Larsen, R.K., Barkley, E.W., and Gallelli, J.F. 1981. "Recommendations for the safe handling of injectable antineoplastic drug products." *Am. J. Hosp. Pharm.* 38:1693-5.

Index